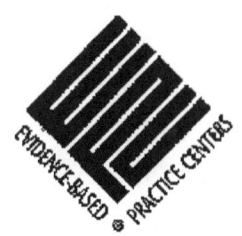

Assessment on Implantable Defibrillators and the Evidence for Primary Prevention of Sudden Cardiac Death

Technology Assessment Report

Project ID: CRDT0511

June 26, 2013

Tufts Evidence-based Practice Center

Katrin Uhlig, M.D., M.S.
Ethan M. Balk, M.D., M.P.H
Amy Earley, B.S.
Rebecca Persson, B.A.
Ann C. Garlitski, M.D.
Minghua Chen, M.D., M.P.H.
Jenny L. Lamont, M.S.
Michael Miligkos, M.D.
Esther E. Avendano, B.A.

This report is based on research conducted by the Tufts Evidence-based Practice Center under contract to the Agency for Healthcare Research and Quality (AHRQ), Rockville, MD (Contract No. 290 2007 10055 I). The findings and conclusions in this document are those of the author(s) who are responsible for its contents; the findings and conclusions do not necessarily represent the views of AHRQ. No statement in this article should be construed as an official position of the Agency for Healthcare Research and Quality or of the U.S. Department of Health and Human Services.

The information in this report is intended to help health care decision-makers; patients and clinicians, health system leaders, and policymakers, make well-informed decisions and thereby improve the quality of health care services. This report is not intended to be a substitute for the application of clinical judgment. Decisions concerning the provision of clinical care should consider this report in the same way as any medical reference and in conjunction with all other pertinent information, i.e., in the context of available resources and circumstances presented by individual patients.

This report may be used, in whole or in part, as the basis for development of clinical practice guidelines and other quality enhancement tools, or as a basis for reimbursement and coverage policies. AHRQ or U.S. Department of Health and Human Services endorsement of such derivative products may not be stated or implied.

This document is in the public domain and may be used and reprinted without special permission. Citation of the source is appreciated.

Persons using assistive technology may not be able to fully access information in this report. For assistance contact TAP@ahrq.hhs.gov.

None of the investigators has any affiliations or financial involvement related to the material presented in this report.

Suggested citation: Uhlig K, Balk EM, Earley A, Persson R, Garlitski AC, Chen M, Lamont JL, Miligkos M, Avendano EE. Assessment on Implantable Defibrillators and the Evidence for Primary Prevention of Sudden Cardiac Death. Evidence Report/Technology Assessment. No. <#>. (Prepared by the Tufts Evidence-based Practice Center under Contract No. 290-2007-10055-I.) Rockville, MD: Agency for Healthcare Research and Quality. June 2013. www.effectivehealthcare.gov/reports/final.cfm.

Preface

The Agency for Healthcare Research and Quality (AHRQ), through its Evidence-based Practice Centers (EPCs), sponsors the development of evidence reports and technology assessments to assist public- and private-sector organizations in their efforts to improve the quality of health care in the United States. The reports and assessments provide organizations with comprehensive, science-based information on common, costly medical conditions, and new health care technologies and strategies.

The EPCs systematically review the relevant scientific literature on topics assigned to them by AHRQ and conduct additional analyses when appropriate prior to developing their reports and assessments. To bring the broadest range of experts into the development of evidence reports and health technology assessments, AHRQ encourages the EPCs to form partnerships and enter into collaborations with other medical and research organizations. The EPCs work with these partner organizations to ensure that the evidence reports and technology assessments they produce will become building blocks for health care quality improvement projects throughout the Nation. The reports undergo peer review and public comment prior to their release as a final report.

AHRQ expects that the EPC evidence reports and technology assessments will inform individual health plans, providers, and purchasers as well as the health care system as a whole by providing important information to help improve health care quality.

We welcome comments on this evidence report. Comments may be sent by mail to the Task Order Officer named in this report to: Agency for Healthcare Research and Quality, 540 Gaither Road, Rockville, MD 20850, or by e-mail to epc@ahrq.hhs.gov.

Carolyn M. Clancy, M.D.
Director
Agency for Healthcare Research and Quality

Jean Slutsky, P.A., M.S.P.H.
Director, Center for Outcomes and Evidence
Agency for Healthcare Research and Quality

Stephanie Chang, M.D., M.P.H.
Director
Evidence-based Practice Program
Center for Outcomes and Evidence
Agency for Healthcare Research and Quality

Kim Marie Wittenberg, M.A.
Task Order Officer
Center for Outcomes and Evidence
Agency for Healthcare Research and Quality

Peer Reviewers

We wish to acknowledge individuals listed below for their review of this report. This report has been reviewed in draft form by individuals chosen for their expertise and diverse perspectives. The purpose of the review was to provide candid, objective, and critical comments for consideration by the EPC in preparation of the final report. Synthesis of the scientific literature presented here does not necessarily represent the views of individual reviewers.

Robin Boineau, MD, MA
Medical Officer
National Heart, Lung, and Blood
Institute
National Institutes of Health
Bethesda, Maryland

Paul Heidenreich, MD, MS
Professor of Medicine
Stanford University
Palo Alto, California

Rita F. Redberg, MD, MSc
Professor of Medicine
UCSF Medical Center
San Francisco, California

Lynne Warner Stevenson, MD
Director Cardiomyopathy/Heart Failure
Program
Professor of Medicine
Brigham and Women's Hospital
Harvard Medical School
Boston, Massachusetts

Ralph J. Verdino, MD
Associate Professor of Medicine
University of Pennsylvania
Philadelphia, Pennsylvania

Assessment on Implantable Defibrillators and the Evidence for Primary Prevention of Sudden Cardiac Death

Structured Abstract

Background: Implantable cardioverter–defibrillators (ICDs) are battery-powered implantable devices that monitor heart rhythm and deliver therapy in the form of either electric shock or antitachycardia pacing (ATP) when a life-threatening ventricular arrhythmia is detected. ICDs have been used in patients who survived sustained ventricular arrhythmias to prevent sudden cardiac death (SCD). In recent years, ICDs have also been implanted for primary prevention (prevention of SCD in a patient who has not had yet had sustained ventricular tachyarrhythmia but has risk factors for it). ICDs may also include cardiac resynchronization therapy (CRT) for additional treatment of heart failure in patients with dyssynchronous ventricles.

Objectives: We aimed to examine the clinical effectiveness of ICD use for primary prevention of SCD. Key Question 1 examined ICD versus no ICD, ICD with ATP versus ICD alone, or ICD with CRT versus ICD alone, and differences among subgroups. Key Question 2 examined early and late adverse events and inappropriate shocks after ICD implantation, and differences among subgroups. Key Question 3 examined eligibility criteria and evaluation methods for patients included in comparative studies and the risk of SCD.

Data Sources: MEDLINE® (through December 4, 2012) and the Cochrane Central Trials Registry (through the third quarter of 2012), with no language exclusion.

Review Methods: For Key Questions 1 and 3, we included comparative studies of ICDs for primary prevention. For Key Question 2, we examined reports from ICD registries or other cohort studies with at least 500 patients with ICDs for primary or secondary prevention. Details on design, patients, interventions, outcomes and quality were extracted into standard forms.

Results: There were 14 studies comparing ICD versus no ICD, 3 studies comparing ICD with CRT (CRT-D) versus ICD, and 59 articles contributing data on adverse events after ICD implantation. There is a high strength of evidence for benefit from ICD treatment compared to control treatment without an ICD for reducing all cause mortality. Meta-analysis of seven RCTs comparing ICD versus control yielded a summary hazard ratio (HR) of 0.69 (95% confidence interval [CI] 0.60, 0.79) for death favoring ICD treatment. Across RCTs, the number needed to treat (NNT) to prevent one death ranged from 6.2 (95% CI 4.0, 18) to 22 (95% CI 2.3, infinite) at the longest durations of followup (3 to 7 years). There is a high strength of evidence for benefit from ICD treatment compared to control treatment without an ICD for reducing SCD. Meta-analysis of five studies comparing ICD versus control showed benefit from ICD use for reducing SCD (HR 0.37; 95% CI 0.26, 0.52). Across RCTs, the NNT to prevent one arrhythmic death ranged from about 2 to 3 (approximate 95% CI 1.3, 16) to 11 (95% CI 1.3, infinite). Three other trials in which ICDs were implanted immediately after myocardial infarction (MI) or at the time of coronary artery bypass grafting did not show a benefit for all-cause mortality, but two of the trials did show a reduction in SCD. Three RCTs of ICD versus no ICD provided low strength of evidence that failed to show a consistent effect of ICD placement on quality of life.

Analyses failed to show statistically significant differences for all-cause mortality or SCD across subgroups by age, sex, and other patient characteristics; however, there may be an indication that ICDs are more effective in patients with more distant coronary revascularization compared with recent surgery. Studies of patients with recent MIs (within 31 or 40 days) had no reduction in all-cause mortality in contrast with studies in patients with more distant MIs. Due to discordant findings among studies, there is insufficient evidence from four RCTs regarding the relative effect on all-cause mortality among patients who receive CRT-D compared to those who receive ICD alone. Heart failure outcomes and related quality of life measures were not reviewed.

Eligibility criteria were reviewed to assess applicability. Comparative studies included individuals with ischemic or nonischemic dilated cardiomyopathy, and left ventricular ejection fraction was ≤35 percent in all but one study. Eligibility criteria regarding heart failure class were variable. The trials of CRT-D used QRS interval data for eligibility; most other trials did not. Most of the RCTs of ICD tested all patients for nonsustained VT, but with different diagnostic tools. Only one RCT reported performing electrophysiology testing in all patients. Only 4 of the 13 RCTs explicitly tested for coronary stenosis, mostly with coronary angiography or exercise testing. Most studies excluded older adults over 70 to 80 years. SCD occurred in 4 to 13 percent of control patients during the 2 to 5 years after randomization.

A high strength of evidence shows early (in-hospital) adverse event rates of approximately 3 percent and serious adverse event rates of approximately 1 percent. Low strength of evidence shows variable, late (out of hospital) rates for device- and lead-related adverse events. Moderate strength evidence shows 3 to 21 percent of patients experience at least one inappropriate shock over 1 to 5 years of followup.

Limitations of the evidence base in some RCTs include lack of blinding of outcome assessors of arrhythmia outcomes or SCD, high attrition rates (>20%), or differential rates of attrition or crossover between study groups and differences in the control treatments or in the rates of concomitant use of beta blockers between the study groups. Nonsignificant findings in subgroup analyses need to be interpreted in the context of studies likely being underpowered to explore differences in effects across subgroups of interest. The quality of the long-term adverse events suffered from a lack of harmonized definitions and systematic ascertainment.

Future research is needed to address comparative effectiveness for quality of life and other patient reported outcomes and to explore treatment heterogeneity according to baseline risk. Consistent reporting of rates of SCD in the non-ICD trial arms would facilitate an assessment of how the mortality benefit may be correlated with the baseline risk.

Conclusions: There is a high strength of evidence that ICD therapy for primary prevention of SCD, versus no ICD therapy, shows benefit with regard to all cause mortality and SCD in patients with reduced left ventricular ejection fraction and ischemic or nonischemic cardiomyopathy beyond the immediate post-MI or coronary revascularization periods. Studies failed to show statistically significant differences for all-cause mortality across subgroups. There is insufficient evidence for all-cause mortality for patients who receive CRT-Ds versus ICD alone for primary prevention. There is high strength of evidence that in-hospital adverse events are infrequent (1-3%) and moderate strength of evidence that up to one-fifth of patients receive inappropriate shocks from the ICDs.

Contents

Tables

Figures

Appendixes

Introduction

Background

Sudden cardiac death (SCD) is the most common cause of cardiovascular death worldwide, accounting for approximately 300,000 deaths in the United States annually, although estimates have ranged from 200,000 to 450,000 deaths.[1-10] The estimate of prevalence depends on the definition and inclusion criteria used in studies.[6] Operationally, SCD is most frequently defined as a cardiac death that occurred within 1 hour of cardiac symptom onset and without another probable cause of death. Studies from epidemiological cohorts from the 1970s through the 1990s suggest that 88 to 91 percent of deaths that occur within 1 hour of symptom onset are arrhythmic in nature.[11] The temporal definition of SCD strongly influences epidemiological data.[6,12] Increasing the time window to 24 hour since symptom onset to define SCD increases the sensitivity but reduces specificity by reducing the proportion of all sudden natural deaths that are due to cardiac causes.

Approximately three-quarters of cases of SCD are caused by ventricular tachyarrhythmias such as ventricular tachycardia (VT) and ventricular fibrillation (VF).[2,13,14] Sustained ventricular arrhythmias may lead to hemodynamic instability and abrupt loss of consciousness without spontaneous recovery, requiring cardiac resuscitation (i.e., cardiac arrest). With advancements in cardiopulmonary resuscitation and greater availability of automatic external defibrillators, it is possible to "abort" SCD. Nonetheless, only 3 to 10 percent of patients who have an out-of-hospital cardiac arrest are successfully resuscitated.[15] Timely administration of therapy is essential, as the rate of survival for people with VF declines by approximately 10 percent per minute.[5,16] Even for those out-of-hospital arrests who survive to hospitalization, survival to hospital discharge is less than 8 percent.[5,17,18]

Prevention is the primary strategy to lower death from SCD. However, SCD is a particular management challenge because the majority of cases occur in individuals without a prior diagnosis of cardiac disease or other clear risk factors for SCD. The most common underlying cardiovascular diagnosis among people with SCD is coronary artery disease (CAD). Yet, in about half of the cases of SCD, SCD itself is the initial manifestation of CAD.[1,4-6] The clinical strategy to prevent death from SCD involves identification of risk factors for ventricular tachyarrhythmias and SCD, to target individuals for medical and interventional treatments.

Outcomes Adjudication

There is the potential to misclassify SCD; thus, to interpret trial results, it is important that studies clearly define their primary and secondary outcomes and follow rigorous methods of adjudication. The most unambiguous outcome with regard to classification is death from any cause or total mortality; this is therefore a common outcome. Arguably, all-cause death is the principal outcome of interest to patients and their families, even though the goal of ICD implantation is to prevent specifically SCD or death from arrhythmia. SCD is a common secondary outcome in ICD trials. However, determination of cause-specific mortality may be fraught with errors. From the Framingham Heart Study, it is suggested that SCD rates derived from death certificates alone should be interpreted with caution.[19] In clinical trials, adjudication of arrhythmia or SCD can be very involved requiring validation by blinded committees which independently adjudicate all deaths according to algorithms and consensus

Criteria for adjudication of SCD were originally developed by Hinkle and Thaler[20] and previously validated in the Canadian Implantable Defibrillator Study[21] and the Canadian Amiodarone Myocardial Infarction Arrhythmia Trial.[22] These criteria are based on the clinical circumstances of death and do not rely on ICD information. Documentation of the cause of death may further incorporate information obtained from witnesses, relatives and family members, death certificates, hospital records, and autopsy reports where available.

Risk Factors for SCD

Risk factors for SCD are multifactorial, dynamic, and associated with a continuous risk function.[23] Some risk factors are nonmodifiable, such as sex and family history of CAD.[24] The incidence of SCD increases as a function of advancing age. The incidence is 100-fold less in young adults less than 30 years of age as compared with older adults.[6,25-28] In regard to the development of disease processes, the Framingham Heart Study revealed that CAD is associated with a 2.8- to 5.3-fold increase in risk of SCD. Following myocardial infarction, there is a 4-fold higher risk of SCD for women and a 10-fold higher risk of SCD for men.[11] Mortality following ST-segment elevation myocardial infarction (MI), in particular, is high with an especially high risk of SCD in those patients with left ventricle dysfunction in the first 30 days.[29] Modifiable CAD risk factors that have been demonstrated to predict SCD include hypertension, hypercholesterolemia, and diabetes.[11] In regard to hypertension which is both an established risk factor for CAD and SCD, both the electrocardiogram pattern of left ventricular hypertrophy and echocardiographic evidence of left ventricular hypertrophy are associated with a higher proportion of sudden and unexpected cardiac death.[6] There are also meaningful associations between cigarette smoking, obesity, lifestyle and SCD. For instance, in a study of 310 survivors of out-of-hospital cardiac arrest, the recurrent cardiac arrest rate was 27 percent at 3 years of follow-up among those who continued to smoke as compared with 19 percent in those who stopped.[30]

The Framingham Heart Study also showed that congestive heart failure is associated with a 2.6- to 6.2-fold increased risk of SCD.[11,31] Other disease processes that impart a variable risk of SCD are cardiomyopathies such as dilated, hypertrophic, and arrhythmogenic right ventricular cardiomyopathy as well as primary electrical disorders such as long QT syndrome and Brugada syndrome. Population-based studies have demonstrated that electrocardiography criteria such as an elevated resting heart rate,[32] prolonged QRS duration,[33,34] and prolonged QT interval increase SCD risk in the general population.[11,35,36]

Currently, the single most widely used risk stratification criterion, based on multiple randomized controlled trials, is a reduced left ventricular ejection fraction (LVEF), typically a value of ≤30 or ≤35 percent.[23] From a pathophysiologic standpoint, the presence of scar tissue is known to be a substrate for ventricular tachyarrhythmias. Molecular, cellular and interstitial changes play a role in myocardial remodeling. One of the challenges of better risk stratification is the fact that different pathophysiological processes may lead to ventricular tachyarrhythmias and subsequently SCD. Thus, the predilection toward a ventricular arrhythmia is complex and cannot be entirely defined by a single dichotomous variable such as LVEF. Further, the greatest absolute number of SCD events will occur in people without known risk factors or with SCD as the first manifestation of cardiac disease.[14,37] In one study which examined patients who had a cardiac arrest, approximately 65 percent would not have qualified for a primary prevention ICD prior to the event.[38] Thus, there is a great need for improved risk stratification tools. Attempts have been made to calculate SCD risk score models such as one derived from Multicenter Automatic Defibrillator Implantation Trial (MADIT)II as well as the Duke risk score in patients with coronary artery disease. The risk scores may be helpful in guiding therapy for a physician but they have not been applied in a prospective manner in clinical trials.[39,40]

An example of an invasive risk stratification tool which has been studied prospectively in Multicenter Unsustained Tachycardia Trial (MUSTT)[41] and MADIT[42] is the electrophysiology study. MUSTT provided evidence that electrophysiologically guided antiarrhythmic therapy with ICDs reduces the risk of SCD in high-risk patients with CAD, LVEF ≤40 percent, spontaneous and unsustained VT, or sustained tachyarrhythmia induced by programmed stimulation. MADIT[42] included patients with CAD and a prior MI, LVEF ≤35 percent, and inducible, sustained VT or VF at electrophysiologic study.[42] Thus, the electrophysiology study has a tailored role in risk prediction.

Medical and Interventional Treatment for Prevention of SCD

Prevention strategies include risk factor modification and treatment of the underlying disease processes of CAD, congestive heart failure, and cardiomyopathy with medical therapy. Medical therapy includes the use of aspirin, beta blockers, angiotensin converting enzyme inhibitors, angiotensin receptor blockers, aldosterone blockers, and statins. In addition, reperfusion therapies for MI such as tissue plasminogen activators and percutaneous coronary intervention for CAD have resulted in a significant decline in SCD over the past 30 years.[43]

Antiarrhythmic drugs have also been used in an attempt to lower the risk of SCD. These medications can effectively suppress abnormal rhythms; however, suppression of arrhythmias with these drugs has not been found to translate into improved survival. In fact these medications have no effect or can increase the risk of SCD. The Cardiac Arrhythmia Suppression Trial (CAST) showed that suppression of spontaneous ventricular arrhythmias with antiarrhythmic agents in high-risk patients after MI resulted in an excess mortality.[44,45] Studies of other antiarrhythmic drugs such as D-sotalol[46] and dronedarone[47] have also resulted in mortality concerns. Amiodarone has not been associated with improved survival in high-risk patients after MI (in two trials, European Myocardial Infarction Amiodarone Trial [EMIAT][48] and Canadian Amiodarone Myocardial Infarction Arrhythmia Trial [CAMIAT],[22] nor has it resulted in improved survival when compared to an implantable cardioverter–defibrillator (ICD) in patients who had a prior cardiac arrest (in the Cardiac Arrest Study Hamburg [CASH],[49] Canadian Implantable Defibrillator Study [CIDS],[21] and Antiarrhythmics versus Implantable Defibrillators [AVID][50] trials). The Sudden Cardiac Death in Heart Failure Trial (SCD-HeFT) showed no survival benefit from amiodarone for primary prevention of SCD when compared with placebo.[51] Furthermore, the use of amiodarone can cause long-term harms involving lung, liver, thyroid, and skin. Given the excess adverse events from antiarrhythmic therapy, antiarrhythmic drugs currently are only selectively administered in some patients to reduce symptoms from recurrent ventricular arrhythmias, without the intention to improve mortality.

In this setting of inadequate medical treatment of ventricular tachyarrhythmias, another treatment option is device therapy. In 1980, Mirowski et al. developed a paradigm of interventional treatment with the development of the ICD,[52] a medical device designed to prevent SCD by terminating ventricular tachyarrhythmias and subsequently aborting cardiovascular collapse and death.

ICD Technology

The ICD is a battery-powered implantable device that consists of a generator and one or more leads capable of sensing a ventricular arrhythmia and delivering therapy in the form of an electric shock. This electric shock causes defibrillation when a potentially life-threatening arrhythmia is detected, to terminate the arrhythmia and prevent SCD. Over the years, ICD technology has evolved in several ways. Over time, the size of the device, or footprint, has become significantly smaller. With improved technology, large abdominal generators have been replaced by smaller pectoral generators. Furthermore, the ICD lead was initially designed as an epicardial patch, which required opening the chest for surgical implantation. At present, right atrial, right ventricular, and left ventricular leads may all be placed endocardially via a transvenous approach, obviating the need for thoracotomy or sternotomy in most cases.

Over the past decade, there has also been an evolution in ICD technology. ICDs were initially designed as single chamber devices with the sole purpose of providing an electric shock to terminate a lethal ventricular rhythm. These devices can now incorporate pacing capabilities to provide backup ventricular pacing. A dual chamber device (with a lead in the right atrium and a lead in the right ventricle) may be implanted to impart atrial and ventricular synchrony in patients who meet indications for a dual chamber pacemaker (i.e., those with certain types of bradycardia) as well as defibrillator therapy.

Currently, device-based therapy also includes the ability to deliver cardiac resynchronization therapy (CRT) via the addition of a left ventricular lead. CRT may be delivered in the form of a standalone biventricular pacemaker (CRT-P) or in addition to an implantable cardioverter defibrillator (CRT-D). CRT implantation involves the placement of right atrial, right ventricular, and left ventricular leads. The difference between CRT-P and CRT-D relates to the type of right ventricular lead (with or without coils) and the type of generator. The goal of CRT is to improve cardiac output in patients who manifest electrical dyssynchrony and cardiac dysfunction via atrial-synchronized biventricular pacing towards improving congestive heart failure and related symptoms as well as prolonging survival. While patients at increased risk for SCD and those who have dyssynchrony share some characteristics, they are not exactly the same clinical populations. The goals of ICD and CRT therapy overlap in their overall goal to improve meaningful survival, but they are distinct in that the intention of ICD therapy is restoration of normal sinus rhythm in the setting of life-threatening arrhythmias, and the intention of CRT is improvement of functional status and symptoms of heart failure.

Technological advances have taken place not only in the design of the generator and the leads but also in software algorithms. One of the goals of these algorithms is to avoid "inappropriate" shocks, shocks that are delivered when ventricular tachyarrhythmias are not occurring. This can occur when there is a fast rhythm that is actually supraventricular (atrial) in origin rather than ventricular. To prevent these inappropriate shocks, ICD programming has been developed to discriminate among types of tachyarrhythmias and to differentiate atrial from ventricular arrhythmias. An inappropriate shock may also be delivered as a result of electromagnetic interference or a lead or device malfunction.

Further developments that combine pacing capabilities with sophisticated programming algorithms include the ability to treat ventricular tachycardias via antitachycardia pacing (ATP). ATP is achieved by pacing the ventricle at a cycle length faster than the ventricular tachyarrhythmia in an attempt to abort the rhythm. Because ICD shocks are painful and are associated with patient morbidity,[53-55] ATP offers the potential to terminate the abnormal rhythm in a painless manner without the need for an electrical shock. On the other hand, ATP may accelerate a VT resulting in the degeneration of the rhythm into VF. The safety and efficacy of ATP has been evaluated in multiple studies.[56-59] Most recently, MADIT-RIT (Multicenter

Automatic Defibrillator Implantation Trial: Reduce Inappropriate Therapy) examined effect of ICD programming on inappropriate therapy and mortality.[60]

ICD Complications

Any potential benefits have to be balanced against potential harms. Implantating a cardiac electronic device is an invasive procedure with inherent risks. There is the potential for intraoperative or immediate postoperative complications, including but not limited to bleeding, infection, pneumothorax, cardiac tamponade, or lead dislodgement.[61-65] Long-term complications include lead or generator malfunction, thrombosis of the access site, infection, and inappropriate ICD shocks that may have emotional and psychological repercussions. In addition to patient characteristics, physician characteristics such as training and volume may play a role in complications rates.[66,67]

ICD Use for Secondary Prevention of SCD

Persons with sustained VT and survivors of out-of-hospital cardiac arrest have an actuarial incidence of SCD at 2 years of 15 to 30 percent.[11,68] Initial use and testing of ICDs was performed in this group of patients who had already experienced a sustained ventricular tachyarrhythmia or SCD and were at high risk of recurrence. This scenario of preventing SCD recurrence is called secondary prevention of SCD. A meta-analysis of three randomized controlled trials (CASH,[49] CIDS,[21] and AVID[50]) of antiarrhythmic therapy versus ICD in this population revealed a 28 percent reduction in the relative risk of death with the ICD.

The current 2008 joint American College of Cardiology Foundation/American Heart Association guidelines for device-based therapy state that ICD therapy is indicated in patients who are survivors of cardiac arrest due to VF or hemodynamically unstable sustained ventricular tachyarrhythmia following exclusion of completely reversible causes.[69]

ICD Use for Primary Prevention of SCD

ICDs have begun to be used in patients with no prior episode of sustained ventricular tachyarrhythmia or SCD but who are considered to be at high risk for SCD. As noted above, the majority of cases of SCD occur in people with no known history of VT or VF. Thus, primary prevention (i.e., preventing a first occurrence) of SCD is of paramount importance.

Current Guidelines

In 2008, a joint task force of the American College of Cardiology Foundation (ACCF)/American Heart Association (AHA)/Heart Rhythm Society in collaboration with the American Association for Thoracic Surgery and Society of Thoracic Cardiac Pacemakers and Antiarrhythmia Devices updated the 2002 guidelines for device-based therapy.[2,70] According to these clinical guidelines, class I indications for ICD therapy for primary prevention of SCD include 1) Patients with LVEF ≤35 percent due to prior MI who are at least 40 days post-MI and are in NYHA Class II or III; 2) Patients with nonischemic dilated cardiomyopathy who have an LVEF ≤35 and who are in NYHA Class II or III. 3) Patients with LV dysfunction due to prior MI who are at least 40 days post-MI, have an LVEF ≤30 percent, and are in NYHA Class I.[70] These clinical indications correlate with the coverage criteria set by CMS.

This review is focused on primary prevention of SCD and does not provide a comprehensive assessment of the effectiveness of CRT for management of heart failure or dyssynchrony.

However, given overlapping indications for CRT and ICD therapy, it is important to note that in October 2012, a joint ACCF/AHA task force on practice guidelines published a focused update, revising its 2008 guidelines.[71] Recommendations specifically for CRT were updated on the basis of multiple heart failure trials in the 2012 Focused Update for Device-Based Therapy of Cardiac Rhythm Abnormalities; ACC/AHA Guidelines for the Management of Patients with Heart Failure; and ICD Indications.[72-74] New recommendations and modifications focused on heart failure status, QRS duration, left versus non-left bundle branch block, and underlying rhythm (sinus rhythm vs. atrial fibrillation). In addition, the Appropriate Use Criteria have been published based on a 2013 HRS-ACC-AHA Expert Consensus on ICD Indications Outside of Current Guidelines.[75] This document assessed levels of appropriateness for implanting ICDs and CRTs in 369 real-life case scenarios, to provide guidance concerning the decision to implant ICDs and CRT devices in a variety of clinical scenarios where there are gaps in guidelines. The AUC document should be used in conjunction with the ACC/AHA/HRS 2008 Guidelines for Device-Based Therapy of Cardiac Rhythm Abnormalities and the 2012 Focused Update.

CMS Coverage Decisions for Primary Prevention

CMS issued coverage decisions for ICD implantation for primary prevention which are reviewed here since they have shaped subsequent research and clinical care. In 2003, CMS provided coverage for primary prevention of SCD, primarily on the basis of data from the Multicenter Automatic Defibrillator Implantation Trial (MADIT)[42]—which included patients with CAD and a prior MI, LVEF ≤35 percent, and inducible, sustained VT or VF at electrophysiologic study—and from MADIT II[76]—which included patients with prior MI and, LVEF ≤30 percent.

The 2005 CMS national coverage determination broadened the indications for implantation of ICDs for primary prevention of SCD.[77] In addition to the above criteria, it added the following indications:

- Documented prior MI and a LVEF ≤30 percent
- Ischemic dilated cardiomyopathy, prior MI, New York Heart Association (NYHA) class II or III heart failure, and LVEF ≤35 percent
- Current CMS coverage requirements for a CRT device, together with ambulatory NYHA class IV heart failure
- Nonischemic dilated cardiomyopathy for >3 months, NYHA class II or III heart failure, and LVEF ≤35 percent.

To be covered, a patient must also be receiving optimal medical therapy and have reasonable expectation of survival with good functional capacity for more than 1 year.

As part of its coverage determination, Medicare instituted a requirement for the CMS to establish an ICD registry to collect data on individuals undergoing ICD implantation to be able to assess outcomes after ICD implantation. Thus, the National Cardiovascular Data Registry (NCDR) ICD registry has been active since 2005.

Current Uncertainties

The field of ICD implantation for primary prevention of SCD is evolving as clinicians are challenged by decisions about how to direct it to patients who may derive net benefit. A number of recent developments may have impacted the risk benefit ratio. With the 2005 coverage decision, the pool of patients eligible for implantation has expanded. Selection criteria have changed with earlier trials selecting patients based on invasive electrophysiological testing, while more recent studies selected patients solely based on clinical selection criteria. Meanwhile, technology has advanced to newer generations of devices. While the risk of SCD is highest in the first few weeks after MI in patients with left ventricular dysfunction, there has been a decrease in the SCD and mortality after MI as a result of medical and percutaneous coronary interventional advances.[29,43] This highlights the need for an updated evaluation of the aggregate data on ICD benefits and harms and how they apply to particular patient subgroups.

Aim of the Technology Assessment

This Technology Assessment examines the state of evidence related to ICD use for primary prevention of SCD. It examines the effectiveness of treatment with an ICD versus control treatment without an ICD. It also examines the effectiveness of combining an ICD with ATP or with CRT versus an ICD alone.

Key Questions

This Technology Assessment considers evidence regarding the following three Key Questions, based on those originally drafted by CMS and refined through discussions with the Agency for Healthcare Research and Quality (AHRQ) and CMS:

Key Question 1

a) In candidates for ICD implantation for primary prevention of SCD, what are the effects of ICD compared with no ICD therapy on clinical outcomes and patient-reported outcomes?
b) In candidates for ICD implantation for primary prevention of SCD, what are the effects of ICD with ATP versus ICD alone, or of ICD with CRT versus ICD alone on clinical outcomes and patient-reported outcomes?
c) How do outcomes vary within the following subgroups?
  i. Different patient characteristics such as varying demographic features, major comorbidities, different risk factors for SCD, or different indications for ICD implantation
  ii. Different ICD characteristics
  iii. Different characteristics of clinicians implanting ICDs—that is, different levels of training and experience
  iv. Different characteristics of facilities where ICDs are implanted

Key Question 2

a) What are the adverse events related to treatment with an ICD for primary prevention of SCD? Specifically:
  i. Early (during hospitalization for implantation)
  ii. Late
  iii. Inappropriate shocks
b) How do adverse events vary within the following subgroups?
  i. Different patient characteristics such as varying demographic features and major comorbidities
  ii. Different ICD characteristics

    iii. Different characteristics of clinicians implanting ICDs—that is, different levels of training and experience

    iv. Different characteristics of facilities where ICDs are implanted

Key Question 3

Which patients have been included in comparative studies of ICDs for primary prevention of SCD?

a) What were eligibility criteria for patients in studies included for Key Question 1? How were patients evaluated and what diagnostic tests and algorithms were used to select patients?

b) Among patients in studies included for Key Question 1, what was the likelihood of SCD or ventricular tachyarrhythmia, as measured by total shocks for those with ICDs or episodes of SCD for those without ICDs?

Methods

The methods for this Technology Assessment follow the AHRQ *Methods Guide for Effectiveness and Comparative Effectiveness Reviews* (hereafter referred to as the Methods Guide; available at www.effectivehealthcare.ahrq.gov/methodsguide.cfm).[78]

AHRQ Task Order Officer

The AHRQ Task Order Officer (TOO) was responsible for overseeing all aspects of this project. The TOO facilitated a common understanding among all parties involved in the project, resolved ambiguities, and fielded all EPC queries regarding the scope and processes of the project. The TOO and other staff at AHRQ reviewed the report for consistency, clarity, and to ensure that it conforms to AHRQ standards.

External Expert Input

The Coverage and Analysis Group at the Centers for Medicare and Medicaid Services (CMS) requested this report from The Technology Assessment Program (TAP) at the Agency for Healthcare Research and Quality (AHRQ). AHRQ assigned this report to the Tufts Evidence-based Practice Center: (Contract Number: 290 2007 10055 I).

The Key Questions in this TA were drafted by CMS and refined by the Evidence-based Practice Center (EPC) through discussions with Agency for Healthcare Research and Quality (AHRQ) Task Order Officer and CMS experts

Key Questions

Key Questions were refined to take into account the patient populations, interventions, comparators, outcomes, and study designs that are clinically relevant for the use of ICDs in the primary prevention of SCD. Three Key Questions are addressed in the present report. Key Question 1 pertains to clinical outcomes (benefits) of ICDs for primary prevention of SCD. Key Question 2 pertains to adverse events associated with ICDs. Key Question 3 pertains to the description of patients enrolled in ICD trials for primary prevention. The Key Questions are listed at the end of the Introduction.

Analytic Framework

To guide the development of the Key Questions for the evaluation of ICDs, we developed an analytic framework (**Figure 1**) that maps the specific linkages associating the populations of interest, the interventions, and the outcomes of interest (intermediate outcomes, surrogate outcomes, and clinical outcomes). Specifically, this analytic framework depicts the chain of logic that evidence must support to link the interventions to improved health outcomes.

Figure 1. Analytic framework for the evaluation of ICDs in the primary prevention of SCD

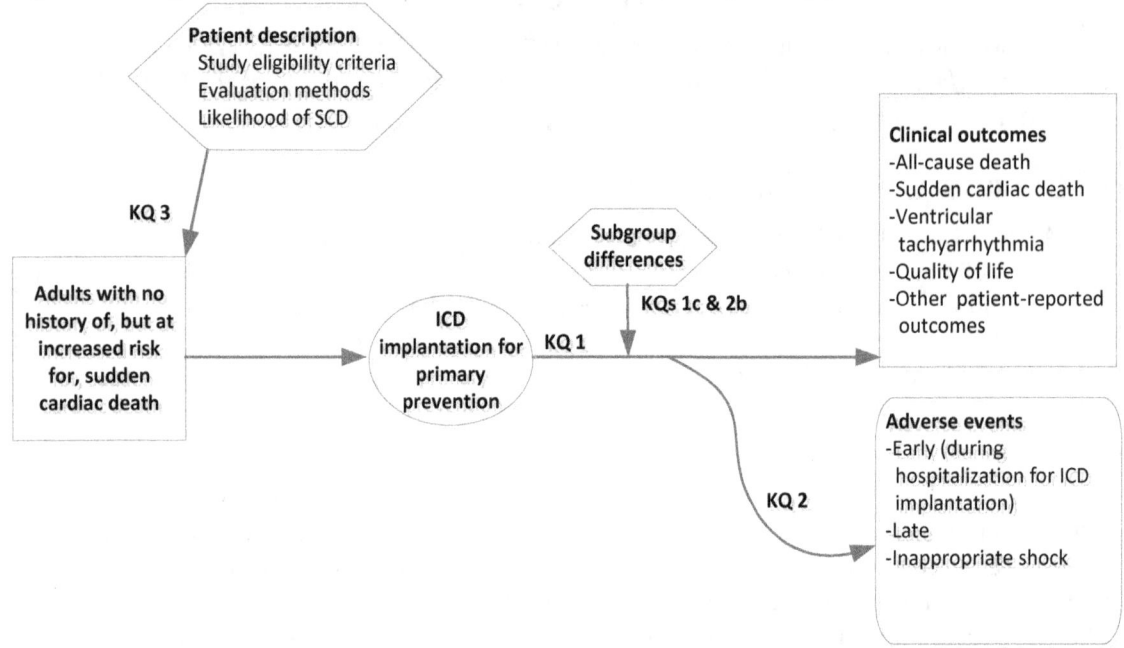

The Key Questions (KQs) are shown within the context of the PICO (Population, Intervention, Comparators, and Outcomes) criteria. The figure illustrates how implantable cardioverter–defibrillator (ICD) implantation for primary prevention of sudden cardiac death affects clinical outcomes and may result in adverse events.

Literature Search and Study Selection

We conducted the literature search in MEDLINE® and the Cochrane Central Register of Controlled Trials with no language restrictions (**Appendix A**). Key words included terms related to the device of interest (ICDs) and terms related to study design. The first search was performed on November 11, 2011, with a final update on December 4, 2012.

Key Question 1

For Key Question 1, randomized controlled trials (RCTs) or comparative longitudinal cohort studies (nonrandomized comparative studies [nRCSs]) were eligible if they provided relevant data directly comparing an ICD to no ICD, including antiarrhythmic drug treatment, or to different ICD interventions and if they included at least 10 participants per study group. For nRCSs, only those studies that used concurrent controls and reported a multivariate analysis were included. The population of interest included adults potentially eligible to receive an ICD for primary prevention of SCD (i.e., adults with no known history of SCD or ventricular tachyarrhythmia). If the study included patients receiving ICDs for secondary prevention, the articles had to provide results by subgroups or specify that the proportion of secondary prevention was less than 20 percent. Participants had to be followed from the time of ICD implantation, not only from some arbitrary time after ICD implantation. There was no minimum followup duration.

For Key Question 1a, comparisons of interest were ICD versus no ICD (i.e., medical management with a designated comparator drug or with concomitant medical therapy). For this review, we included studies comparing CRT-D versus CRT alone as a comparison of ICD versus no ICD. For Key Question 1b, comparisons of interest were ICD with ATP versus ICD alone, or ICD with CRT CRT versus ICD versus ICD alone. We did not review comparisons of different pacing or shock algorithms.

For Key Question 1c, we examined effect modification in subgroups. In studies eligible for Key Questions 1a and 1b, we examined the results across subgroups for different patient characteristics such as varying demographic features (age, sex, race, and ethnicity), major comorbidities, different risk factors for SCD, or different indications for ICD implantation (including LVEF$\geq$30 versus < 30 percent, duration of QRS interval, NYHA heart failure classification, and type of underlying heart disease [e.g., ischemic vs. nonischemic cardiomyopathy]); time from MI; different numbers of leads; different characteristics of clinicians implanting ICDs—that is, different levels of training and experience; and different characteristics of facilities where ICDs are implanted, such as patient volume and presence or absence of a training program. We planned to evaluate subgroups that were of particular interest to CMS upon setting up the ICD registry: patients with LVEF of 31 to 35 percent, patients with nonischemic cardiomyopathy of less than 9 months' duration, and patients with NYHA class IV heart failure who may benefit from an ICD with CRT. Studies had to report how a difference in the factor affected outcomes of interest (e.g., death rates in subgroups based on age ranges), not the groups' baseline characteristics on the basis of the outcome (e.g., mean ages at ICD implantation among patients who survived or died). We examined whether estimates differed statistically significantly across subgroups.

For all of Key Question 1, outcomes of interest were clinical outcomes including death from SCD, all-cause mortality, sustained ventricular tachyarrhythmia, quality of life (QoL), and other patient-reported outcomes. We excluded heart failure outcomes as well as composite outcomes of death and heart failure. For QoL and other patient-reported outcomes, we gave priority to measurements made with standardized and validated instruments.

Key Question 2

For rates of adverse events, we included longitudinal studies of any design with at least 500 participants. This criterion was set because the rate of adverse events is low and because we were able to use a registry for in-hospital adverse events. Participants had to be followed from the time of ICD implantation, not only from some arbitrary time after ICD implantation. There was no minimum followup duration. For comparison of rates of different ICD devices we reviewed comparative studies with at least 10 patients per arm that were included in Key Question 1b.

The population of interest was adults who received an ICD for primary prevention alone, preferentially, or for either primary or secondary prevention, if not separately reported. A mix of primary and secondary prevention was permitted because we determined that there is little reason to expect adverse events to differ between primary prevention and secondary prevention populations and that the addition of patients with ICDs for secondary prevention would allow for better estimates of adverse event rates. However, studies specifying ICD implantation only for secondary prevention were excluded. We also excluded studies published prior to 2002, because we aimed to focus on harms associated with current devices and implantation methods.

Interventions of interest were the same as those for Key Question 1: single-chamber, dual-chamber, or biventricular ICDs with or without ATP or CRT. The outcomes of interest for adverse events are listed below, divided into those that occur early after ICD implantation (including events that occur during the hospital stay for implantation or up to 30 days postimplantation) and those occurring later:

- Early (during hospitalization for ICD implantation)
  - Any adverse event
  - Any adverse event or death
  - Any serious adverse event
  - Atrioventricular fistula
  - Cardiac arrest
  - Cardiac perforation
  - Cardiac valve injury
  - Cerebrovascular accident/Stroke
  - Conduction block
  - Coronary venous dissection
  - Drug reaction
  - Hematoma
  - Hemothorax
  - Infection related to device
  - Lead dislodgement
  - Myocardial infarction
  - Pericardial tamponade
  - Peripheral embolism
  - Peripheral nerve injury
  - Phlebitis - deep
  - Phlebitis - superficial
  - Pneumothorax
  - Transient ischemic attack
- Late (after hospitalization for implantation)
  - Device malfunction
  - Device or lead revision
  - Lead dislodgement
  - Lead fracture or malfunction
  - Infection related to device
  - Thrombosis
- Inappropriate shocks

For adverse events occurring early after the implantation procedure (during hospitalization), we reviewed and reconciled reports from the NCDR ICD database. This registry was started after the 2005 Medicare coverage decision and provides standardized, comprehensive data on over 90 percent of ICD implantations in the United States with active and passive ascertainment for adverse events during the hospitalization for the implantation.[79] We included all pertinent reports from the registry even though there was overlap in participants across publications.

For adverse events occurring after hospitalization, we included cohort studies with ICD groups, including ICD arms from RCTs. Since the adverse events of interest are unique to the ICD or the implantation procedure, we did not extract data on control arms without ICDs. For information on how adverse events differ across ICD types, we tabulated the adverse events reported in eligible comparative studies from Key Question 2.

We further searched for any information on effect modifiers that might increase or decrease the risk of adverse events. Subgroups or factors of interest were different patient characteristics (age, sex, race, diabetes, end-stage renal disease), different ICD characteristics (including ATP or CRT features and number of leads), different characteristics of clinicians implanting the ICDs (different levels of training and experience), and different characteristics of facilities where ICDs are implanted. For subgroups, we again included only data reported on the basis of the factor, not on the basis of the outcome, and examined whether estimates differed statistically significantly across subgroups.

Key Question 3

For Key Question 3a, related to the eligibility criteria and prior evaluation of participants, we reviewed the studies used to address Key Question 1 and tabulated the descriptive information about how patients were evaluated prior to enrollment and randomization. For Key Question 3b, we evaluated the studies reviewed for Key Question 1 and captured the number of total shocks and ATP pacing events as an indicator of the underlying severity of disease (i.e., the likelihood of SCD) in patients analyzed in studies to assess treatment heterogeneity across studies. Note that the number of inappropriate shocks, a measure of harm, is covered in Key Question 2.

Article Screening and Data Extraction

We screened titles and abstracts using *Abstrackr* (http://sunfire34.eecs.tufts.edu).[80] Seven researchers double-screened the abstracts after iterative training of all reviewers on several batches of abstracts. Discordant decisions and queries were resolved at group meetings. Full-text articles were retrieved for all potentially relevant abstracts. Studies excluded during full-text screening and the reasons for exclusion are given in **Appendix B**.

Each study was extracted by one experienced methodologist. The extraction for results and quality were reviewed and confirmed by at least one other methodologist. Data extraction was done using the Systematic Review Data Repository (SRDR) database (www.srdr.ahrq.gov).[81] The form was customized to capture all relevant elements for the key question and included elements for population characteristics, sample size, study design, descriptions of the ICD and comparison interventions, outcomes, subgroup factors, and relevant results analyses. We also extracted data on items of particular relevance to Key Question 3, such as eligibility criteria and how patients were evaluated.

For data from survival curves, we extracted both the reported hazard ratio (HR), preferentially the adjusted HR rather than the unadjusted HR, and any reported counts data. We did not digitize figures to estimate counts or percentages of outcomes. We used the maximum duration of the survival curve as the duration of followup for each relevant outcome, unless the article explicitly expressed the HR as applying to a different timepoint. For outcomes with data reported at multiple timepoints, our *a priori* timepoints of interest for clinical outcomes were 1, 2, and 4 years of followup. In our meta-analyses (described below), we also analyzed data from all years of followup with data.

Risk of Bias and Quality of Reporting Assessment

For Key Question 1, we assessed methodological quality of RCTs using eight items derived from the Cochrane risk of bias tool[82] and one additional item created to address participant crossovers during the study period (**Table 1**). Reviewing across all eight risk of bias items, we assigned an overall quality grade of good, fair, or poor to each RCT. We assigned particular weight to risk of bias concerns related to differential attrition or crossover between arms and to differences other than ICD assignment between the two arms. We downgraded for risk of bias related to outcome assessor blinding only for clinical outcomes other than all-cause mortality. We did not grade nonrandomized comparative studies (nRCS).

For Key Question 2, we assessed the quality of reporting of harms using items adapted from the McMaster Quality Assessment Scale of Harms (McHarm) Tool (**Table 2**).[83,84]

Table 1. Risk of bias items assessed for randomized controlled trials (Key Question 1)

1. What is the risk of selection bias (biased allocation to interventions) due to inadequate generation of a randomized sequence?
2. What is the risk of selection bias (biased allocation of interventions) due to inadequate concealment of allocations before assignment?
3. For each main outcome or class of outcomes, what was the risk of detection bias due to knowledge of the allocated interventions by outcome assessment (lack of outcome assessor blinding)?
4. For each main outcome or class of outcomes, what is the risk of attrition bias due to amount, nature, or handling of incomplete outcome data?
5. Were all randomized participants analyzed in the group to which they were allocated?
6. Were the groups similar at baseline regarding the most important prognostic indicators?
7. Were co-interventions avoided or similar?
8. Are there other risks of bias? If yes, describe them in Notes.
9. Number of crossovers?

Table 2. Quality of reporting items assessed for adverse event studies (Key Question 2)

1. Were any harms pre-specified (*a priori*) in methods section?
    1a. If yes, were any of them pre-specified with *a priori* standardized or precise definitions?
2. Were all pre-specified harms reported?
3. Was the mode of harms collection active (sought to collect information on adverse events)?
4. Was the mode of harms collection passive? (Participants are not specifically asked about or tested for the occurrence of adverse events. Rather, adverse events are identified based on patient reports made on their own initiative.)
5. Did the study specify the timing and/or frequency of collection of harms?
6. Is the number of participants who experience harms provided for each arm?
7. Is the number at risk for harms (denominator) provided for each arm?
8. For comparative studies (those also addressing Key Question 1): Is there statistical analysis of relative harms between groups?

Data Synthesis

We summarized all included studies in narrative form as well as in evidence tables that summarize the important features of the study design, population characteristics, results, study quality, and inclusion criteria. Tables in **Appendix C** provide detailed baseline characteristics of the included patients and cointerventions given at baseline, the qualitative results summary, the quality of each study, and the results for Key Question 3 (See Table of Contents for Appendix C).

For outcomes with at least three RCTs with sufficiently similar comparisons of interventions and comparators (relevant to Key Question 1), we performed DerSimonian & Laird random effects model meta-analyses.[85] We meta-analyzed adjusted HRs, unadjusted HRs (if no adjusted HR was reported), and estimated HRs (if no HR was reported). To estimate the HR, we used the various methods described by Tierney et al. to estimate HR given different types of reported data.[86] For these calculations, only reported counts (events) were used; we did not use digitized data from figures. For each meta-analysis the statistical heterogeneity was assessed with the I^2 statistic, which describes the percentage of variation across studies that is due to heterogeneity rather than chance.[87,88]

For our primary meta-analyses, we included only studies that included only patients who meet current practice for ICD use for primary prevention, thus excluding studies of patients undergoing ICD implantation immediately after coronary revascularization or early after recent myocardial infarction. We conducted sensitivity analyses in which we added back in the RCTs of these "atypical" patients.

To assess how the effect of ICD versus no ICD changes over time since randomization we drew plots of the difference in cumulative mortality between ICD and no ICD based on the reported Kaplan Meier plots for each trial. At each year timepoint we estimated the cumulative death proportion by digitizing the figure for both ICD and no ICD and subtracted the no ICD cumulative death proportion from the ICD proportion. This calculation measures the vertical distance between the two curves in the Kaplan Meier plots. To roughly estimate the average difference in cumulative death across studies we calculated a weighted mean of the differences at each annual time point based on the numbers of people remaining at risk within each study at each timepoint.

For each RCT of ICD versus no ICD, we calculated the numbers-needed-to-treat (NNT) to prevent one death (all-cause) and to prevent one tacchyarrhythmia death. Since most RCTs reported HRs for death, we estimated the NNT for each trial to prevent one death at each year from reported or estimated HRs. To estimate NNT from HR, we used the method described by Altman et al., which estimates the control and treatment rates from the HR, the survival rate at each year, and the number at risk at each year.[89] Since the control rates across studies varied widely, we did not meta-analyze NNT as the summary NNT value would be uninterpretable without a single value for the control rate as a referent.

In regards to subgroup analyses, for each study that reported odds ratios (or relative risks or hazard ratios) for the same or similar pairs of subgroups (e.g., women vs. men, age≤60 or 65 years vs. >60 or 65 years), we calculated a "relative odds ratio" as the ratio of the odds ratio (or similar metric) of one subgroup to the other subgroup, and its 95 percent confidence interval. When at least three studies reported sufficient data for pairs of similar subgroups, we meta-analyzed these using a random effects model.

Strength of Evidence Grading

We followed the Methods Guide to evaluate the strength of the body of evidence for Key Questions 1 and 2 with respect to four domains: risk of bias, consistency, directness, and precision.[78,90] Briefly, we defined the risk of bias (low, medium, or high) on the basis of the study design and the methodological quality of the studies. Where there was sufficient evidence from RCTs, we determined strength of evidence from these alone, without considering the nRCSs.

For consistency we did not use rigid counts of studies as standards of evaluation (e.g., four of five studies agree, therefore the data are consistent); instead, we assessed the direction, magnitude, and statistical significance of all studies for each specific topic and made a qualitative determination.

Since we examined clinical and patient-reported outcomes (and clinically important adverse events), we expected all analyzed evidence to be "direct." Where applicable, we considered the degree to which conclusions are based on direct comparisons (within studies) or indirect comparisons across studies).

We assessed the precision of the evidence as precise or imprecise on the basis of the degree of certainty surrounding each effect estimate. A precise estimate is one that allows for a clinically useful conclusion. An imprecise estimate is one for which the confidence interval is wide enough to include clinically distinct conclusions (e.g., both clinically important superiority and inferiority—a situation in which the direction of effect is unknown) and that therefore precludes a conclusion.

We rated the body of evidence on the basis of four strength-of-evidence levels (high, moderate, low, and insufficient[90]) to indicate our level of confidence that the evidence reflects the true effect for the major comparisons of interest.

A high strength of evidence suggests that we are very confident that the estimate of effect lies close to the true effect for this outcome. The body of evidence has few or no deficiencies. We believe that the findings are stable.

A moderate strength of evidence suggests that we are moderately confident that the estimate of effect lies close to the true effect for this outcome. The body of evidence has some deficiencies. We believe that the findings are likely to be stable, but some doubt remains.

A low strength of evidence suggests that we have limited confidence that the estimate of effect lies close to the true effect for this outcome. The body of evidence has major or numerous deficiencies (or both). We believe that additional evidence is needed before concluding either that the findings are stable or that the estimate of effect is close to the true effect.

A ranking of insufficient evidence suggests that we have no evidence, we are unable to estimate an effect, or we have no confidence in the estimate of effect for this outcome. No evidence is available or the body of evidence has unacceptable deficiencies, precluding judgment. We graded the body of evidence to be insufficient to assess a strength of evidence if evidence was either unavailable or did not permit estimation of an effect because of lacking or sparse data or if the data were too inconsistent or inconclusive to determine whether there was evidence of a benefit, a harm, or no difference between intervention and comparator. In general, when only one study had been published, the evidence was considered insufficient, unless the study was particularly large, robust, and of good quality.

We reviewed subgroups results for Key Question 1 and 2 for statistically significant differences. Subgroup analyses are by their nature exploratory. Thus we did not grade strength of evidence of the subgroup results.

Applicability

We followed the Methods Guide to evaluate the applicability of included studies to patient populations of interest.[78,90] We highlighted limitations to applicability when comparing the populations in the included studies with the core Medicare population.

Peer Review

The draft report was prereviewed by the AHRQ TOO. Following revisions, the draft report was sent to invited peer reviewers and simultaneously uploaded to the AHRQ Web site where it was available for public comment for 2 weeks. All reviewer comments (both invited and from the public) were collated and individually addressed. The revised report and the EPC's responses to invited and public reviewers' comments were again reviewed by the TOO prior to completion

16

of the report. The authors of the report had final discretion as to how the report was revised on the basis of the reviewer comments, with oversight by the TOO.

Results

Our searches identified a total of 10,866 abstracts, of which we screened 348 in full text and included 84 articles (**Figure 2**). **Appendix B** lists the studies that were excluded in full text. There were 31 articles that described 13 randomized controlled trials (RCTs) and 4 nonrandomized comparative studies (nRCSs) that address Key Questions 1 and 3. For Key Question 2, there were 59 articles that included 37 independent study cohorts of patients with ICD, including 4 RCTs that compared different types of ICDs. Six articles (Five studies) were included in both Key Questions 1 and 2.

Figure 2. Literature Flow Diagram

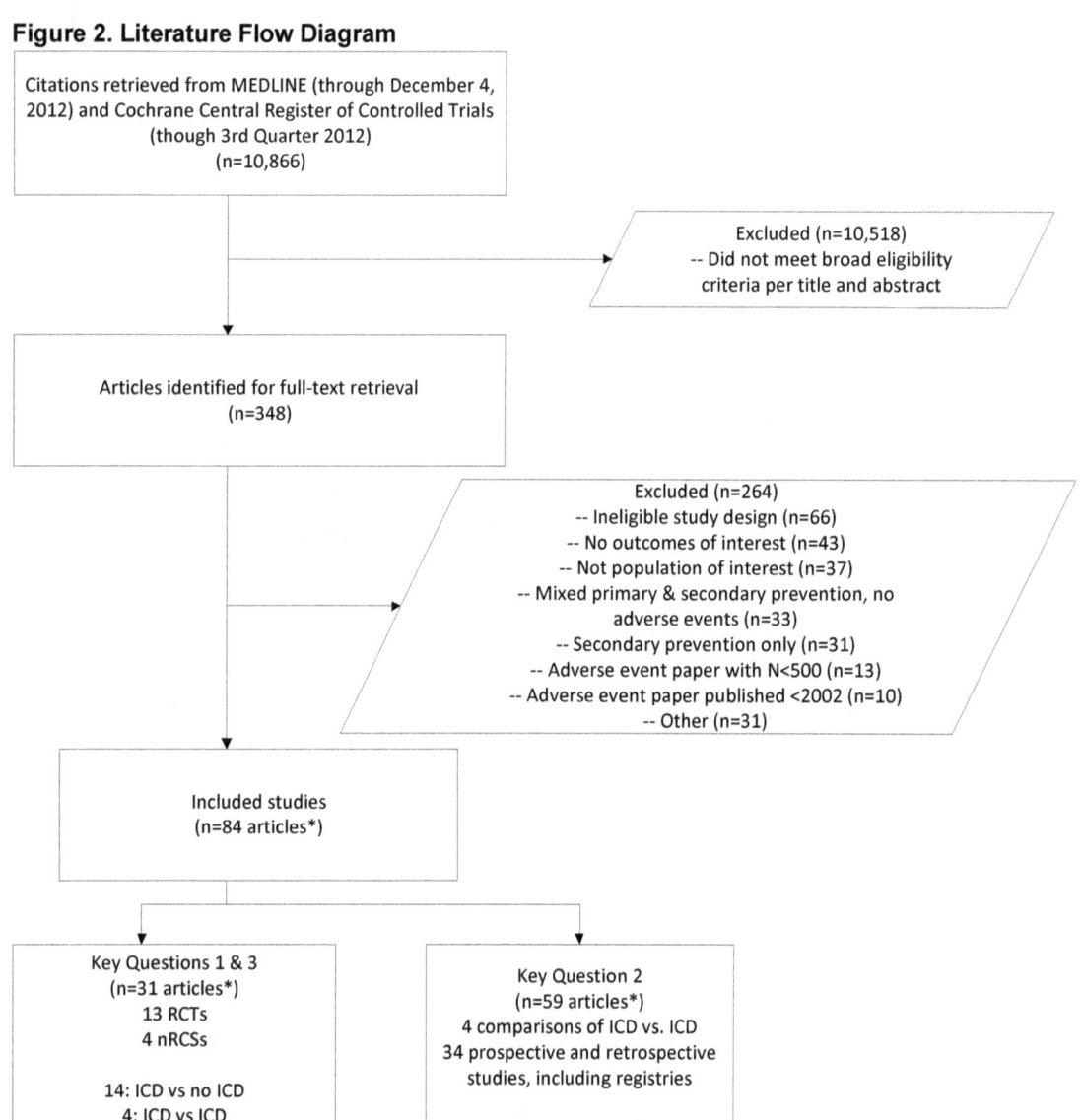

ICD = implanted cardioverter defibrillator, nRCSs = nonrandomized comparative studies, RCTs = randomized controlled trials. Studies could have had more than one reason for exclusion but only one reason for each is listed here.
* Includes multiple publications (articles) derived from the same studies. Five articles on 4 studies provided data for Key Questions 1 and 2.

Of note, under Key Question 1, we have incorporated Key Question 1c (on subgroups) into both Key Questions 1a (ICD vs. no ICD) and 1b (ICD vs. ICD).

The list following this paragraph includes all studies included for Key Question 1, with their acronyms defined. In the Discussion section, we explain why several well-known ICD trials did not meet eligibility criteria.

AMIOVERT	Amiodarone Versus Implantable Cardioverter-Defibrillator: Randomized Trial in Patients With Nonischemic Dilated Cardiomyopathy and Asymptomatic Nonsustained Ventricular Tachycardia
CABG-Patch	Coronary Artery Bypass Graft Patch Trial
CAT	Cardiomyopathy Trial
Chan 2009	
COMPANION	Comparison of Medical Therapy, Pacing and Defibrillation in Heart Failure
DEFINITE	Defibrillators in Nonischemic Cardiomyopathy Treatment Evaluation
Diab 2011	
DINAMIT	Defibrillator in Acute Myocardial Infarction Trial
Fonarow 2000	
IRIS	Immediate Risk Stratification Improves Survival
MADIT	Multicenter Automatic Defibrillator Implantation Trial
MADIT II	Multicenter Automatic Defibrillator Implantation Trial II
MADIT-CRT	Multicenter Automatic Defibrillator Implantation Trial with Cardiac Resynchronization Therapy
MENDMI	Prevention of Myocardial Enlargement and Dilation Post Myocardial Infarction Study
Mezu 2011	
OPTIMIZE-HF/GWTG-HF	Organized Program to Initiate Lifesaving Treatment in Hospitalized Patients with Heart Failure and Get With the Guidelines-Heart Failure
RAFT	Resynchronization-Defibrillation for Ambulatory Heart Failure
SCD-HeFT	Sudden Cardiac Death in Heart Failure Trial

Key Questions 1a & 1c:
In Candidates for ICD Implantation for Primary Prevention of SCD, What Are the Effects of ICD Therapy Compared with No ICD Therapy on Clinical Outcomes and Patient-Reported Outcomes? How Do Outcomes Vary Within Subgroups?

For Key Questions 1a and 1c, we included studies that compared ICD use with no ICD use, with or without concomitant CRT or ATP in adults being treated for primary prevention of SCD. Except as noted, we did not distinguish between studies that compared ICD with no ICD (both arms with or without antiarrhythmic drugs) and studies that compared ICD alone with antiarrhythmic drugs. The findings and strength of evidence for outcomes with sufficient evidence for the comparison of ICD versus no ICD are summarized in **Table 3**.

Table 3. Summary of findings for ICD vs. no ICD

Outcome	Study Design: No. Studies (N)	Findings	Strength of Evidence
All-cause mortality	ICD vs. no ICD RCT: 10 (8,606) nRCS: 4 (5,949)	• ICD use as primary prevention for patients who meet the current practice criteria (no recent MI, no concurrent coronary revascularization) reduces the risk of all-cause mortality over the course of 3 to 7 years after implantation: HR = 0.69 (95% CI 0.60, 0.79). The benefit of ICD appears fairly stable over time. Across trials, the range of NNT to prevent one death was 6.2 to 22 at 3 to 7 years, with wide 95% CIs. • There is indirect evidence across studies that patients with recent MIs (<30-40 days), on average, do not benefit from ICD, in contrast with patients with more distant MIs. • Within-study subgroup analyses fail to support whether the value of ICD placement differs in other subgroups of patients, including by sex or age, or based on different characteristics of facilities where ICDs are implanted.	High
Sudden cardiac death	ICD vs. no ICD RCT: 7 (4,093) nRCS: 2 (1,115)	• ICD use as primary prevention for patients who meet the current practice criteria (no recent MI, no concurrent coronary revascularization) reduces the risk of SCD over the course of 2 to 6 years after implantation: HR = 0.37 (95% CI 0.26, 0.52). There is insufficient evidence to evaluate the course of the effect over time. Across trials, the range of NNT to prevent one SCD was approximately 2.0 to 11. • Within-study subgroup analyses fail to support whether the value of ICD placement differs in subgroups of patients or based on different characteristics of facilities where ICDs are implanted.	High
Quality of life	ICD vs. no ICD RCT: 3 (1,825)	• The evidence fails to show a consistent effect of ICD placement on quality of life. • There is no evidence regarding subgroups.	Low

CI = confidence interval, CMS = Centers for Medicare and Medicaid Services, HR = hazard ratio, ICD = implantable cardioverter–defibrillator, MI = myocardial infarction, NNT = number-needed-to-treat, No. = number, nRCS = nonrandomized comparative study, RCT = randomized, controlled trial, SCD = sudden cardiac death.

We identified 10 RCTs (reported in 18 articles[42,51,76,91-104]) and 4 nRCSs[105-108] (**Table 4**). Among the 14 RCTs, 9 were assessed to be of good quality and 5 of fair quality (**Figure 3, Appendix Table 8**); 2 of these trials were further downgraded (to fair or poor quality) for outcomes other than all-cause mortality because outcome assessors were not blinded.[92,94] Methodological concerns included high attrition rates (>20%),[95] differential rates of attrition and/or crossover between study groups,[51,94,95,99] and differences in the rates of use of beta blockers between the two study groups.[51] Of note, all trials conducted intention-to-treat analyses.

We did not explicitly grade the methodological quality of the four nRCSs, though we included only studies that performed multivariable analyses.

The 14 studies were published from 1996 to 2011 and the patients' mean ages ranged from 48 to 86 years. The RCTs enrolled between 103 and 2,521 patients, and the nRCSs analyzed between 147 and 4,685 patients. The majority of patients in these studies were men with LVEF ranging from 21 to 28 percent. All four New York Heart Association (NYHA) classes were represented in the study samples. Two studies (one RCT[95] and one nRCS[106]) included only patients with NYHA Class III or IV heart failure. The RCT enrolled approximately 84 percent Class III patients and the nRCS enrolled half Class III and half Class IV patients. The percentage of patients with diabetes ranged widely across the studies, from 5 to 63 percent. Additional information about the characteristics of the patients included in the studies is described under Key Question 3.

Of note, two of the trials that met eligibility criteria (IRIS and DINAMIT)[98,102] included patients who would not meet current CMS criteria for an ICD because they were restricted to patients who had a recent MI (within 31 or 40 days). In a third trial, CABG-Patch,[94] ICD implantation took place at the time of coronary artery bypass graft (CABG). These patients would also fall outside of the current clinical guidelines for implantation as well as guidelines for CMS coverage. Thus, the primary meta-analyses of the RCTs exclude these three trials, though they are included in tables, forest plots, and sensitivity analyses.

All-Cause Mortality

All 10 RCTs and 4 nRCSs reported data on long-term all-cause mortality (**Appendix Table 3**). We meta-analyzed the RCT data, as shown in **Figure 4**. The studies followed patients for approximately 3 to 7 years (mean followup durations of about 1.3 to 5.5 years). ICD implantation resulted in a lower risk (or hazard) of all-cause death (summary HR 0.69; 95% CI 0.60, 0.79) without statistical heterogeneity. The estimated NNTs to prevent one death for these studies (Table 8) ranged from 6.2 (95% CI 4.0, 18) to 22 (95% CI 2.3, infinite) at the longest durations of followup (3 to 7 years).

It should be noted that two studies—COMPANION[95] and SCD-HeFT[51]—were three-arm studies that each included two non-ICD interventions that could be construed as the comparator of interest. The first study, COMPANION had the following three arms: ICD with CRT (CRT-D), CRT without ICD (CRT-P), and medical therapy. We determined that the medical therapy arm, not the CRT-P arm, was most similar to the comparison arms in other studies. The second study, SCD-HeFT included the following three arms: ICD, medical therapy (not including amiodarone), and medical therapy with amiodarone. The study found no difference in death rates between the amiodarone and no amiodarone groups. We chose the medical therapy without amiodarone as the most relevant control arm.

In sensitivity analyses, including the studies that were the most clinically different from the rest resulted in weaker effect sizes and greater statistical heterogeneity. Including the two studies that included patients with recent MIs (IRIS and DINAMIT) yielded a smaller effect favoring ICD but with statistical heterogeneity (HR 0.76 [95% CI 0.65, 0.91; $I^2 = 44\%$]). Alternatively, including CABG-Patch, which included patients undergoing CABG, yielded a similar effect (HR 0.73 [95% CI 0.62, 0.87; $I^2 = 36\%$]). Including all three atypical studies yielded the smallest effect with the greatest heterogeneity (HR 0.80 [95% CI 0.68, 0.94; $I^2 = 51\%$])

Figure 5 suggests that the reduction in overall mortality imparted by ICD is fairly stable over time from 1 to 7 years. The maximal difference in how many people have died was approximately 10 percent. The MADIT trial may differ from other trials in that the point estimates of the difference in cumulative death was about twice as large favoring ICD than other studies, but again the difference between ICD and no ICD was fairly stable, excluding year 5 when only 3 patients were still at risk of dying in the study (since most patients were not yet followed for that long). As suggested by the wide confidence intervals for HRs of all-cause mortality for MADIT and other trials (Figure 4), the difference between MADIT and the other studies may be due solely to random chance. The results in AMIOVIRT differed in that the benefit of ICD did not appear until year 3. The three atypical studies (CABG-Patch, DINAMIT, and IRIS; shown in grey in Figure 5), by definition consistent with their larger HRs for death compared with other studies, found no sustained benefit of ICD over time (the differences in cumulative death were near zero or positive, indicating fewer deaths with no ICD).

The four nRCSs all examined the effects of ICD versus no ICD on all-cause mortality (**Appendix Table 3**). There was one prospective cohort study and three retrospective cohort studies. The studies varied in duration of followup from 2 to 5 years. All four provided data on all-cause mortality at 2 to 3 years. All found reduced all-cause mortality with ICD implantation versus no ICD. The range of adjusted HRs was 0.46 (95% CI 0.22, 0.98) to 0.78 (95% CI 0.44, 1.30), favoring ICD use. Three of the four studies found the adjusted HRs to be statistically significant.

Two of the trials (MADIT and CABG-Patch) also reported 30-day mortality data (**Appendix Table 6**). MADIT had no deaths in either group at 30 days. CABG-Patch did not report mortality rates, but noted no significant difference in 30-day mortality rates.

Subgroup Data: All-Cause Mortality

Eight RCTs and two nRCSs (17 publications) provided data on the differential effects of ICD placement (versus no ICD) based on 11 different subgroups.[94] **Table 5** presents subgroup data for subgroup variable pairs that were reported by at least two studies, including by sex, age, NYHA Class, LVEF, presence of heart failure, presence of left bundle branch block, QRS duration, time since myocardial infarction, blood urea nitrogen, and diagnosis of diabetes. **Appendix Table 5** is a more complete version of the table, also including subgroup analyses that were reported by unique studies; this table also includes data based on type of heart disease (ischemic versus nonischemic), prior coronary revascularization, time since coronary revascularization, kidney function, and other specific subgroups not included in Table 5.

Among 76 subgroup analyses across the 10 studies, no significant differences were found in relative all-cause mortality between ICD and no ICD groups for subgroup analyses, with the exception of a comparison of NYHA Class II and III patients in SCD-HeFT (ICD effective in patients with Class II heart failure, but not Class III).[51] Meta-analyses the relative OR of death for women vs. men (**Figure 6**), age subgroups (**Figure 7**), LVEF subgroups, QRS duration subgroups, and diabetes vs. no diabetes were all statistically homogeneous and found no significant difference between the respective subgroups.

SCD-HeFT[51] and COMPANION[95] examined time since coronary revascularization and both found greater, but not significantly different, benefits for ICD use in patients with more distant coronary revascularization. In MADIT II, among patients with revascularization >6 months prior HR=0.64 compared with HR=1.19 with more recent revascularization, but P=0.29.[97] SCD-HeFT found that for patients with CABG >2 years prior HR=0.71 compared with HR=1.40 with more recent CABG (P=0.09), but time since percutaneous coronary revascularization was not associated with ICD benefit.[109] An indirect comparison of ISIS and DINAMIT (which included patients with recent MIs, within 31 or 40 days) versus the remaining trials, suggests that patients with recent MIs may have no reduction in all-cause mortality (HR 1.05 [95% CI 0.86, 1.30]) than patients with more distant or no prior MIs (HR 0.69 [95% CI 0.60, 0.79]). By meta-regression, the difference between IRIS and DINAMIT and the other seven RCTs is statistically significant (P = 0.012).

Evaluation across studies for other indirect comparisons of subgroups did not reveal any additional subgroup differences.

Summary: All-Cause Mortality

Ten RCTs of fair to good quality and four nRCSs that directly compared ICD with no ICD (or amiodarone) provided consistent and precise findings of a significant benefit of ICD to reduce all-cause mortality (**Table 7**). There is a high strength of evidence that ICD use as primary prevention for patients who meet the current CMS practice criteria (no recent MI, no concurrent coronary revascularization) reduces the risk of all-cause mortality by about 31 percent (95% CI 21, 40) percent over the course of 3 to 7 years after implantation (**Table 3**). The reduction in all-cause mortality appears fairly stable over time across studies. Across RCTs, the NNT to prevent one death ranged from 6.2 (95% CI 4.0, 18) to 22 (95% CI 2.3, infinite) at the longest durations of followup (3 to 7 years). Overall, within-study analyses failed to show statistically significant differences for all-cause mortality across subgroups; however there may be an indication that ICDs are more effective in patients with more distant coronary revascularization or MIs compared with recent surgery (within either 6 months or 2 years) or MI (within 31 or 40 days). There are no data for different characteristics of clinicians implanting ICDs or facilities where ICDs are implanted.

Sudden Cardiac Death (Arrhythmic Death)

Seven RCTs (six good quality, one fair quality) and two nRCSs reported data on SCD (or death from cardiac arrhythmia) (**Appendix Table 7**). We meta-analyzed the RCT data, as shown in **Figure 7**. The studies followed patients for between 2 and 6 years. In general, SCD event rates were low, such that in four of the six RCTs, three or fewer individuals had SCD in one or both study groups during study followup. In the CAT study,[91] no SCD events occurred at 2 years of followup. Nevertheless, in all studies (except CAT), SCD was less common in patients who had an ICD than those without an ICD. The summary HR across the four primary analysis trials (excluding the atypical studies) was 0.37 (95% CI 0.26, 0.52) with no statistical heterogeneity (I^2 = 0). However, the lack of heterogeneity can largely be ascribed to the wide CIs within each study. Sensitivity analysis including IRIS and DINAMIT yielded a smaller effect size (summary HR 0.241; 95% CI 0.31, 0.54). **Figure 9** suggests that the effect of ICD versus no ICD on SCD proportions over time is fairly stable but may increase beyond 2 or 3 years. Among the four eligible RCTs with adequate data (Table 9), the estimated NNT to prevent one arrhythmic death was 1.9 to 3.2 in three trials (approximate 95% CIs 1.3, 16) and 11 (95% CI 1.3, infinite) in the fourth RCT.

The two nRCSs examined the effects of ICD versus no ICD on SCD (**Appendix Table 7**). Fonarow 2000,[106] a retrospective cohort study, followed patients for 2 years; Chan 2009,[105] a prospective cohort study, followed patients for 3 years. Both found lower risk of SCD with ICD implantation (0 vs. 22% actuarial rate over 2 years, P = 0.05; and adjusted HR = 0.65, 95% CI 0.40, 1.03 over 3 years).

Subgroup Data: Sudden Cardiac Death

Subgroup analyses of SCD-HeFT related to time since MI, prior coronary revascularization, and time since revascularization and subgroup analyses of MADIT II related to time since coronary revascularization and presence of kidney disease all failed to find a significant interaction between ICD placement and subgroups (**Table 6**).[96,97,109,110] No other subgroup analyses have been reported. Indirect comparison across studies fails to show any differences based on patient or other characteristics. There are no data for different characteristics of clinicians implanting ICDs or facilities where ICDs are implanted.

Summary: Sudden Cardiac Death

Seven RCTs of generally good quality and two nRCSs that directly compared ICD with no ICD (or amiodarone) provided consistent and sufficiently precise findings of a significant benefit of ICD to reduce SCD (**Table 7**). There is a high strength of evidence that ICD use as primary prevention for patients who meet the current CMS practice criteria (no recent MI, no concurrent coronary revascularization) reduces the risk of SCD by about 63 percent (95% CI 48, 74) over the course of 2 to 6 years after implantation (**Table 3**). There is a suggestion across studies that the effect of ICD on SCD over time may increase beyond 2 or 3 years. Across RCTs, the NNT to prevent one arrhythmic death ranged from about 2 to 3 (approximate 95% CI 1.3, 16) to 11 (95% CI 1.3, infinite). The evidence fails to support a difference in the benefit of ICD based on time since MI, coronary revascularization, or kidney disease. There is insufficient evidence to evaluate differential effects of ICD on SCD in other subgroups of patients or based on different characteristics of clinicians implanting ICDs or facilities where ICDs are implanted.

Sustained Ventricular Tachyarrhythmia

No study that directly compared ICD to no ICD (or amiodarone) reported on long-term sustained ventricular tachyarrhythmia. The only study to report any data on sustained ventricular tachycardia was CABG-Patch,[100] which reported event rates postoperatively as an adverse event of CABG surgery with or without ICD placement.

Summary: Sustained Ventricular Tachyarrhythmia

There is insufficient evidence to estimate the effect of ICD placement for primary prevention on the rate of sustained ventricular tachyarrhythmia episodes (**Table 7**).

Quality of Life

Three RCTs (two of good quality, 1 fair) reported on the effect of ICD placement versus no ICD placement on various measures of QoL (**Appendix Table 9**). The three trials each evaluated different QoL measures, including the Health Utility Index 3 (MADIT II[101], a health utility assessing health-related QoL across eight attributes: vision, hearing, speech, ambulation, dexterity, emotion, cognition, and pain and discomfort), the Quality of Well-being Schedule (AMIOVIRT[103], assessing both functional and symptom status, translatable into quality-adjusted life years), the State Trait Anxiety Inventory (AMIOVIRT[103], focusing on the anxiety component of QoL), the Short Form 36 (SF-36) (CABG-Patch[100], evaluating eight health concepts: physical functioning, role limitations due to physical problems, bodily pain, general health perceptions, vitality, social functioning, role limitations due to emotional problems, mental health, health transition (perceived change in health), and the Perception of Health Transition scale (CABG-Patch[100], where patients assess their current health status relative to 1 year before). No QoL scale was used by more than a single study.

MADIT II[101] and AMIOVIRT[103] found no statistically significant difference in QoL between ICD and control arms according to the Health Utility Index 3, the State Trait Anxiety Inventory, and the Quality of Well-being Schedule. CABG-Patch,[100] which compared CABG plus ICD placement with CABG without ICD, reported on seven of the SF-36 subscales (not vitality) along with the Perception of Health Transition scale. The trial found no significant difference between the two groups for five of the seven evaluated SF-36 QoL domains, but control patients (those without ICD) reported significantly better QoL for the subscales regarding emotional role functioning and mental health. In addition, control patients had better perception of health transition compared with 1 year prior.

Subgroup Data: Quality of Life

No study reported subgroup analyses for the relative effect of ICD versus no ICD on QoL.

Summary: Quality of Life

Across three RCTs of good and fair quality, only one found that some measures of QoL favored no ICD over ICD (**Table 7**). While the three trials covered a broad range of QoL measures, no specific QoL measure was evaluated by more than a single trial. Furthermore, the single trial that did find a difference (favoring no ICD) for some measures of QoL, is of limited applicability to current practice, both because all patients had CABG and because the trial implanted epicardial ICD systems which are much more invasive and large compared to the transvenous ICDs currently employed. It is unknown to what degree the concurrent CABG or the older technologies may have led to the worse emotional role, mental health, and perception of overall health in those who received ICDs.

Given the sparseness of data on QoL and the lack of consistency across trials, overall, there is a low strength of evidence low strength of evidence that failed to show a consistent effect of ICD placement on QoL (**Table 3**). There is insufficient evidence to evaluate differential effects of ICD on QoL in different populations of patients or based on different characteristics of facilities where ICDs are implanted.

Other Patient-Reported Outcomes

No eligible study reported other patient-reported outcomes of interest. Therefore, there is insufficient evidence to estimate the effect of ICD placement for primary prevention on other patient-reported outcomes (**Table 7**).

Table 4. ICD vs. no ICD: Study characteristics

Study Author Year PMID	Intervention (Control)	NYHA class	Ischemic	Non-ischemic	Non-sustained VT	%LVEF	Total N	Primary outcome	Duration followup	ICD type/No. of leads	Enrollment period
AMIOVIRT Strickberger 2003 12767651	ICD (Amiodarone)	I, II, III	No	Yes	Yes	≤35	103	Death, all-cause	5 y	nd	8/1996-9/2000
CABG-Patch Bigger 1997 9371853	ICD (No ICD)	NYHA not a criterion	Yes	No	No	<36	900	Death, all-cause	4 y mean 32 ± 16 mo (2.67 y)	nd	Pilot began 1990 with full-scale study started in 1993
CAT Bansch 2002 11914254	ICD (Control)	II, III	No	Yes	No	≤30	104	Death, all-cause at 1 y	6 y	nd	5/1991-3/1997
Chan 2009 20031808	ICD (No ICD)	NYHA not a criterion	Yes	Yes	No	≤35	965	Death, all-cause	5 y	nd	3/2001-6/2005
COMPANION Bristow 2004 15152059	ICD + CRT (No ICD)*	III, IV	Yes	Yes	No	≤35	1520	Death from or hospitalization for any cause	1080 d (2.95 y) median 14 mo (weighted average of CRT-D and control groups)	Multi-chamber	1/2000-11/2002
DEFINITE Kadish 2004 15152060	ICD (No ICD)	I, II, III	No	Yes	Yes	<36	458	Death, all-cause	5 y mean 29 ± 14.4 mo (2.42 y)	Single-chamber	1998-2002 (randomization date)
DINAMIT Hohnloser 2004 15590950	ICD (No ICD)	I, II, III	Yes	No	No	≤35	674	Death, all-cause	4 y mean 2.5 y	Single-chamber	1998-nd (last follow-up 9/2003)
Fonarow 2000 10760339	ICD (Control)	III, IV	No	Yes	No	<35	147	nd	mean 22 ± 26 mo	nd	1/1988-1/1997
IRIS Steinbeck 2009 19812399	ICD (No ICD)	I, II, III	Yes	No	Yes	≤40	898	Death, all-cause	6 y mean 37 mo	nd	6/9/1999-10/15/2007

Study Author Year PMID	Intervention (Control)	NYHA class	Ischemic	Non-ischemic	Non-sustained VT	%LVEF	Total N	Primary outcome	Duration followup	ICD type/No. of leads	Enrollment period
MADIT Moss 1996 8960472	ICD (No ICD)	I, II, III	Yes	No	Yes	≤35	196	Death, all-cause	5 y mean 27 mo	Single-chamber	1990-nd (trial stopped in 1996)
MADIT II Moss 2002 11907286	ICD (No ICD)	I, II, III	Yes	No	No	≤30	1232	Death, all-cause	mean 20 mo range 6 d-53 mo	nd	7/11/1997-nd
Mezu 2011 21640321	ICD (No ICD)	I, II, III	Yes	Yes	No	≤35	152	Death, all-cause	4 y mean 2.3 y	nd	1/2000-12/2008
OPTIMIZE-HF and GWTG-HF Hernandez 2010 20009044	ICD (No ICD)	NYHA not a criterion	No	No	No	≤35	4685	Death, all-cause	3 y	nd	2003-2006
SCD-HeFT Bardy 2005 15659722	ICD (no ICD/placebo)#	II or III	Yes	Yes	Yes	≤35	2521	Death, all-cause	6 y median (survivors) 45.5 mo	Single-chamber	9/16/1997-7/18/2001 (randomization date)

*The CRT-P arm of COMPANION study was not used for the meta-analysis

The amiodarone arm of SCD-HeFT was not used for the meta-analysis

AMIOVERT = Amiodarone versus Implantable Cardioverter-Defibrillator Randomized Trial, CABG-Patch = Coronary Artery Bypass Graft Patch, CAT = Cardiomyopathy Trial, COMPANION = Comparison of Medical Therapy, Pacing and Defibrillation in Heart Failure, CRT = cardiac resynchronization therapy, d = day, DEFINITE = Defibrillators in Nonischemic Cardiomyopathy Treatment Evaluation, DINAMIT = Defibrillator in Acute Myocardial Infarction Trial, GWTG-HF = Get With the Guidelines-Heart Failure, ICD = implantable cardiac defibrillator, IRIS = Immediate Risk Stratification Improves Survival, LV = left ventricular, MADIT = Multicenter Automatic Defibrillator Implantation Trial, mo = month, nd = not documented, NYHA = New York Heart Association, OPTIMIZE-HF = Organized Program to Initiate Lifesaving Treatment in Hospitalized Patients with Heart Failure, SCD-HeFT = Sudden Cardiac Death in Heart Failure Trial, VT = ventricular tachycardia, y = year

Table 5 Subgroup analysis data and meta-analyses of ICD vs. no ICD for all-cause death

Study, Author, Year, PMID	Subgroup 1 vs. 2	OR* (CI), Subgroup 1	OR* (CI), Subgroup 2	ROR† (CI)	Reported P‡
Sex					
COMPANION, Bristow, 2004, 15152059	Female vs. Male	0.6 (0.3, 1.1)	0.65 (0.4, 0.9)	0.92 (0.43, 1.99)	nd
DEFINITE, Kadish, 2004, 15152060	Female vs. Male	1.1 (0.5, 2.6)	0.49 (0.27, 0.90)	2.24 (0.81, 6.23)	NS
DINAMIT, Hohnloser, 2004, 15590950	Female vs. Male	1.0 (0.5, 2.1)	1.1 (0.7, 1.7)	0.91 (0.39, 2.11)	0.82
Hernandez, 2010, 20009044	Female vs. Male	0.58 (0.41, 0.83)	0.80 (0.63, 1.01)	0.73 (0.47, 1.11)	0.31
IRIS, Steinbeck, 2009, 19812399	Female vs. Male	1.0 (0.6, 1.7)	1.1 (0.8, 1.5)	0.91 (0.49, 1.67)	0.15
MADIT II, Moss, 2002, 11907286	Female vs. Male	0.6 (0.3, 1.1)	0.7 (0.5, 0.9)	0.86 (0.42, 1.75)	0.85
SCD-HeFT, Russo, 2008 18373605	Female vs. Male	0.90 (0.56, 1.43)	0.71 (0.57, 0.88)	1.27 (0.76, 2.12)	0.54||
CABG-Patch, Bigger, 1997, 9371853	Female vs. Male	nd	nd	nd	NS
MADIT, Moss, 1996, 8960472	Female vs. Male	nd	nd	nd	>0.2
Meta-analysis:	I²=0%			**0.95 (0.75,1.20)**	
Age					
Chan, 2009, 20031808	<65 vs. 65-74 y	0.74 (0.43, 1.28)	0.76 (0.45, 1.29)	0.97 (0.46, 2.08)	0.43¶
COMPANION, Bristow, 2004, 15152059	≤65 vs. >65 y	0.6 (0.3, 0.95)	0.7 (0.5, 1.0)	0.86 (0.44, 1.68)	nd
DEFINITE, Kadish, 2004, 15152060	<65 vs. 65-84 y	0.7 (0.3, 1.4)	0.6 (0.3, 1.2)	1.17 (0.41, 3.29)	NS
DINAMIT, Hohnloser, 2004, 15590950	<60 vs. 60-80 y	0.9 (0.4, 1.9)	1.2 (0.8, 1.9)	0.75 (0.31, 1.83)	0.46
IRIS, Steinbeck, 2009, 19812399	<65 vs. 65-80 y	0.95 (0.6, 1.5)	1.05 (0.8, 1.5)	0.90 (0.52, 1.58)	0.73
MADIT II, Moss, 2002, 11907286	<60 vs. 60-69 y	0.5 (0.2, 0.9)	0.8 (0.5, 1.3)	0.63 (0.26, 1.52)	NS**
SCD-HeFT, Bardy 2005 15659722	<65 vs. ≥65 y	0.68 (0.52, 0.95)	0.86 (0.65, 1.14)	0.79 (0.55, 1.13)	nd
Meta-analysis:	I²=0%			**0.83 (0.66, 1.05)**	
Chan, 2009, 20031808	65-74 vs. ≥75 y	0.76 (0.45, 1.29)	0.59 (0.39, 0.90)	1.29 (0.66, 2.52)	0.43¶
Hernandez, 2010, 20009044	65-74 vs. 75-84 y	0.65 (0.47, 0.89)	0.80 (0.62, 1.03)	0.81 (0.54, 1.22)	0.31
MADIT II, Moss, 2002, 11907286	60-69 vs. ≥70 y	0.8 (0.5, 1.3)	0.6 (0.45, 0.95)	1.33 (0.73, 2.45)	NS**
Meta-analysis:	I²=17%			**1.03 (0.73, 1.45)**	
MADIT, Moss, 1996, 8960472	Age, continuous	--	--	nd	>0.2
CABG-Patch, Bigger, 1997, 9371853	Age, continuous	--	--	nd	NS
NYHA Class					
DEFINITE, Kadish, 2004, 15152060	NYHA Class II vs. III	1.0 (0.5, 2.2)	0.37 (0.15, 0.90)	2.70 (0.85, 8.64)	NS‡‡
SCD-HeFT, Bardy 2005 15659722	NYHA Class II vs. III	0.54 (0.41, 0.81)	1.16 (0.87, 1.44)	0.47 (0.32, 0.67)	<0.001

Study, Author, Year, PMID	Subgroup 1 vs. 2	OR* (CI), Subgroup 1	OR* (CI), Subgroup 2	ROR† (CI)	Reported P‡
Left ventricular ejection fraction					
Chan, 2009, 20031808	LVEF ≤25 vs. 26-35%	0.73 (0.51, 1.04)	0.59 (0.37, 0.93)	1.24 (0.69, 2.22)	0.61
DINAMIT, Hohnloser, 2004, 15590950	LVEF <26 vs. 26-35%	1.5 (0.8, 2.7)	0.85 (0.5, 1.5)	1.76 (0.78, 4.00)	0.16
MADIT II, Moss, 2002, 11907286	LVEF ≤25 vs. 25-30%	0.6 (0.5, 0.9)	0.7 (0.4, 1.2)	0.86 (0.46, 1.60)	NS
Meta-analysis:	**I²=0%**			**1.17 (0.80, 1.70)**	
COMPANION, Bristow, 2004, 15152059	LVEF ≤20 vs. 20-35%	0.6 (0.4, 0.9)	0.7 (0.4, 1.1)	0.86 (0.45, 1.64)	nd
DEFINITE, Kadish, 2004, 15152060	LVEF <20 vs. 20-36%	0.9 (0.4, 2.0)	0.5 (0.3, 0.95)	1.80 (0.67, 4.84)	NS
Heart failure					
CABG-Patch, Bigger, 1997, 9371853	Heart failure vs. No heart failure	nd	nd	nd	NS
Chan, 2009, 20031808	Heart failure vs. No heart failure	0.69 (0.50, 0.93)	0.70 (0.35, 1.41)	0.99 (0.46, 2.11)	0.59
MADIT, Moss, 1996, 8960472	Heart failure vs. No heart failure	nd	nd	nd	>0.2
IRIS, Steinbeck, 2009, 19812399	Heart failure vs. No heart failure	1.0 (0.7, 1.4)	1.2 (0.8, 1.8)	0.83 (0.49, 1.42)	0.56
Left Bundle Branch Block					
COMPANION, Bristow, 2004, 15152059	LBBB vs. No LBBB	0.5 (0.4, 0.8)	0.9 (0.5, 1.6)	0.56 (0.28, 1.09)	nd
MADIT, Moss, 1996, 8960472	LBBB vs. No LBBB	nd	nd	nd	>0.2
MADIT II, Moss, 2002, 11907286	LBBB vs. No LBBB	nd	nd	nd	NS
QRS duration					
DEFINITE, Kadish, 2004, 15152060	QRS <120 vs. ≥120 msec	0.75 (0.4, 1.5)	0.5 (0.2, 1.1)	1.50 (0.51, 4.41)	NS
DINAMIT, Hohnloser, 2004, 15590950	QRS <120 vs. ≥120 msec	0.85 (0.5, 1.4)	1.5 (0.8, 2.9)	0.57 (0.25, 1.29)	0.13
MADIT II, Moss, 2002, 11907286	QRS <120 vs. 120-150 msec	0.7 (0.5, 1.2)	0.6 (0.4, 1.1)	1.17 (0.60, 2.28)	NS††
SCD-HeFT, Bardy 2005 15659722	QRS <120 vs. ≥120 msec	0.84 (0.64, 1.11)	0.67 (0.51, 0.95)	1.25 (0.88, 1.79)	nd
Meta-analysis:	**I²=0%**			**1.13 (0.82, 1.54)**	
Time since Myocardial Infarction					
MADIT II, Wilber, 2004, 14993128	Time since MI <18 vs. 18-51 mo	0.97 (0.51, 1.81)	0.52 (0.26, 1.05)	1.87 (0.73, 4.79)	NS
SCD-HeFT, Piccini, 2011, 21109025	Time since MI <18 vs. 18-59 mo	0.7 (0.37, 1.31)	0.54 (0.3, 0.98)	1.30 (0.55, 3.08)	0.33∥∥
MADIT II, Wilber, 2004, 14993128	Time since MI 18-59 vs. 60-119 mo	0.52 (0.26, 1.05)	0.50 (0.26, 0.91)	1.04 (0.41, 2.66)	nd
SCD-HeFT, Piccini, 2011, 21109025	Time since MI 18-51 vs. 52-111 mo	0.54 (0.3, 0.98)	1.47 (0.75, 2.87)	0.37 (0.15, 0.90)	0.33∥∥
MADIT, Moss, 1996, 8960472	Time since MI <6 vs. ≥6 mo	nd	nd	nd	>0.2
MADIT II, Moss, 2002, 11907286	Time since MI <6 vs. ≥6 mo	nd	nd	nd	NS
Blood Urea Nitrogen					
MADIT, Moss, 1996, 8960472	BUN ≤25 vs. >25 mg/dL	nd	nd	nd	>0.2
MADIT II Moss, 2002, 11907286	BUN ≤25 vs. >25 mg/dL	nd	nd	nd	NS

29

Study, Author, Year, PMID	Subgroup 1 vs. 2	OR* (CI), Subgroup 1	OR* (CI), Subgroup 2	ROR† (CI)	Reported P‡
Diabetes mellitus					
Chan, 2009, 20031808	DM vs. No DM	0.68 (0.45, 1.03)	0.69 (0.48, 1.01)	0.99 (0.56, 1.72)	0.95
DINAMIT, Hohnloser, 2004, 15590950	DM vs. No DM	0.9 (0.5, 1.5)	1.2 (0.8, 2.0)	0.75 (0.37, 1.53)	0.38
SCD-HeFT, Bardy 2005 15659722	DM vs. No DM	0.95 (0.71, 1.24)	0.67 (0.52, 0.93)	1.42 (0.99, 2.03)	nd
CABG-Patch, Bigger, 1997, 9371853	DM vs. No DM	nd	nd	nd	NS
IRIS, Steinbeck, 2009, 19812399	DM vs. No DM	nd	nd	nd	NS
MADIT II, Moss, 2002, 11907286	DM vs. No DM	nd	nd	nd	NS
Meta-analysis:	**I^2=32%**			**1.12 (0.78, 1.61)**	

The table includes only subgroup comparisons for which at least 2 trials reported analyses for similar subgroups. Meta-analyses were performed only if there were at least 3 such studies with sufficient data for a given subgroup comparison.

BUN = blood urea nitrogen, CI = 95% confidence interval, DM = diabetes mellitus, LBBB = left bundle branch block, LVEF = left ventricular ejection fraction, MI = myocardial infarction, nd = no data reported, NS = nonsignificant, NYHA = New York Heart Association, OR = odds ratio, PMID = PubMed ID, ROR = relative odds ratio. See page 16 for study acronyms.

* Reported odds ratio or relative risk or hazard ratio.

† Relative odds ratios and their confidence intervals calculated from reported odds ratios (etc.) for each subgroup.

‡ The reported P value for the interaction among subgroups.

§ OPTIMIZE-HF and GWTG-H

|| For analysis of ICD vs. amiodarone vs. placebo.

¶ For analysis of <65 y vs. 65-74 y vs. ≥75 y.

** For analysis of <60 y vs. 60-69 y vs. ≥70 y

†† For analysis of <120 msec vs. 120-150 msec vs. ≥150 msec.

‡‡ For analysis of NYHA Class I vs. Class II vs. Class III.

|||| For analysis of <18 mo vs. 18-51 mo vs. 52-111 mo vs. >111 mo.

Table 6. Subgroup analyses of ICD vs. no ICD for sudden cardiac death

Study, Author, Year, PMID	Subgroups HR/RR (95% CI)				P Interaction
SCD-HeFT, Piccini, 2011, 21109025	**Time Since MI**				
	<18 mo:	0.47 (0.16, 1.42)	18-51 mo:	0.28 (0.073, 1.10)	P=0.68
	52-111 mo:	0.24 (0.063, 0.89)	>111 mo:	0.25 (0.065, 0.97)	
SCD-HeFT, Al-Khatib 2008, 18479330	**Prior CABG:**	0.52 (0.26, 1.02)	No CABG:	0.44 (0.23, 0.83)	P=0.94
	Prior PCI:	0.31 (0.08, 1.13)	No PCI:	0.51 (0.31, 0.85)	P=0.53
	Time Since CABG:	nd			P=0.38
	Time Since PCI:	nd			P=0.80
MADIT II, Goldenberg, 2006, 16682305	**Time since CR**				
	≤6 mo:	2.01 (0.18, 22.22)	>6 mo:	0.34 (0.19, 0.61)	P=0.16
	7-60 mo:	0.27 (0.11, 0.66)	>60 mo:	0.40 (0.19, 0.86)	nd
MADIT II Goldenberg, 2006, 16893702	**Kidney Disease**				
	eGFR<35:	0.95 (0.23, 4.00)	eGFR ≥35:	0.34 (0.20, 0.56)	P=0.19
	eGFR 35-59:	0.37 (0.19, 0.74)	eGFR≥60:	0.32 (0.15, 0.69)	nd

CABG = coronary artery bypass graft, CI =confidence interval, CR = coronary revascularization, eGFR = estimated glomerular filtration rate (in mL/min/m^2), HR = hazard ratio, ICD = implantable cardiac defibrillator, MI = myocardial infarction, mo = month, nd =no data, PCI = percutaneous coronary revascularization, PMID = PubMed ID, Revasc = revascularization, RR = risk ratio. See page 16 for study acronyms

Table 7. ICD vs. no ICD for primary prevention of SCD: Strength of evidence domains

Outcome	Study Design: No. Studies (N)	Study Limitations	Directness	Consistency	Precision	Reporting Bias	Other Issues	Finding and Strength of Evidence
All-cause mortality (≥1 y)	RCT: 10 (8,606) nRCS: 4 (5,949)*	Low RoB (6 good, 4 fair) Not graded	Direct	Consistent	Precise	Undetected		High ICD reduces all-cause mortality in patients meeting current practice criteria (no recent MI, no concurrent coronary revascularization) HR = 0.69 (95% CI 0.60, 0.79)
All-cause mortality (30 d)	RCT: 2 (1096)	Low RoB (1 good, 1 fair)	Direct	Consistent	Imprecise	Undetected	0 deaths in 1 applicable RCT	Insufficient Unknown difference in 30-day mortality
Sudden cardiac death (arrhythmic death)	RCT: 7 (4,093) nRCS: 2 (1,115)*	Low RoB (6 good, 1 fair) Not graded	Direct	Consistent	Precise	Undetected		High ICD reduces SCD in patients meeting current practice criteria (no recent MI, no concurrent coronary revascularization) HR = 0.24 (95% CI 0.11, 0.56)
Sustained ventricular tachyarrhythmia	0							Insufficient
Quality of life	RCT: 3 (1,825)	Low RoB (2 good, 1 fair)	Direct	Inconsistent	Imprecise	Undetected		Low ICD may not affect quality of life
Other patient-reported outcomes	0							Insufficient

CI = confidence interval, HR = summary hazard ratio, ICD = implanted cardiac defibrillator, nRCS = nonrandomized comparative study, RoB = risk of bias, RCT = randomized controlled trial, SCD = sudden cardiac death.

* The nRCSs are not included in the determination of the strength of evidence

32

Table 8. ICD vs. no ICD: Number-needed-to-treat (95% confidence interval) to prevent one death, by study

Study	Year:	1	2	3	4	5	6	7
MADIT, Moss 1996		3.6	3.7	4.0	4.3	7.2		
8960472		(2.2, 14)	(2.4, 14)	(2.7, 14)	(2.9, 15)	(5.0, 23)		
COMPANION, Bristow 2004		6.4	6.2	6.2				
15152059		(3.8, 20)	(3.9, 18)	(4.0, 18)				
MADIT II, Moss 2002		9.7	7.6	7.4	7.5			
11907286		(4.8, 58)	(4.1, 41)	(4.2, 38)	(4.3, 37)			
DEFINITE, Kadish 2004		9.8	7.2	6.7	6.5	6.4		
15152060		(3.7, inf)	(3.2, inf)	(3.1, inf)	(3.1, inf)	(3.2, inf)		
SCD-HeFT, Bardy 2005		11	12	11	10	10		
15659722		(6.0, 77)	(6.3, 85)	(5.8, 71)	(5.7, 68)	(5.8, 67)		
CAT, Bansch 2002		17	12	8.6	8.4	8.2	8.0	8.1
11914254		(3.5, inf)	(3.0, inf)	(2.6, inf)	(2.6, inf)	(2.6, inf)	(2.8, inf)	(2.9, inf)
AMIOVIRT, Strickberger 2003		29	26	25	22			
12767651		(2.4, inf)	(2.4, inf)	(2.4, inf)	(2.3, inf)			

inf = infinite. See page 16 for study acronyms.

Table 9. ICD vs. no ICD: Number-needed-to-treat (95% confidence interval) to prevent one tachyarrhythmia death, by study*

Study	Year:	1	2	3	4	5
MADIT, Moss 1996			2.0			
8960472			(1.4, 16)			
DEFINITE, Kadish 2004		2.6	2.0	1.9	1.9	1.9
15152060		(1.3, 36)	(1.3, 13)	(1.3, 12)	(1.3, 11)	(1.3, 11)
AMIOVIRT, Strickberger 2003			11			
12767651			(1.3, inf)			
SCD-HeFT, Bardy 2005		4.2	3.5	3.4	3.2	3.2
15659722		(2.6, 9.1)	(2.3, 6.9)	(2.3, 6.4)	(2.3, 6.0)	(2.2, 5.8)

inf = infinite. See page 16 for study acronyms.

* There were no tachyarrhythmia deaths in CAT by 2 years, therefore this study is not included.

Figure 3. Risk of bias for 13 RCTs of ICD vs. no ICD or vs. other ICD for primary prevention of SCD

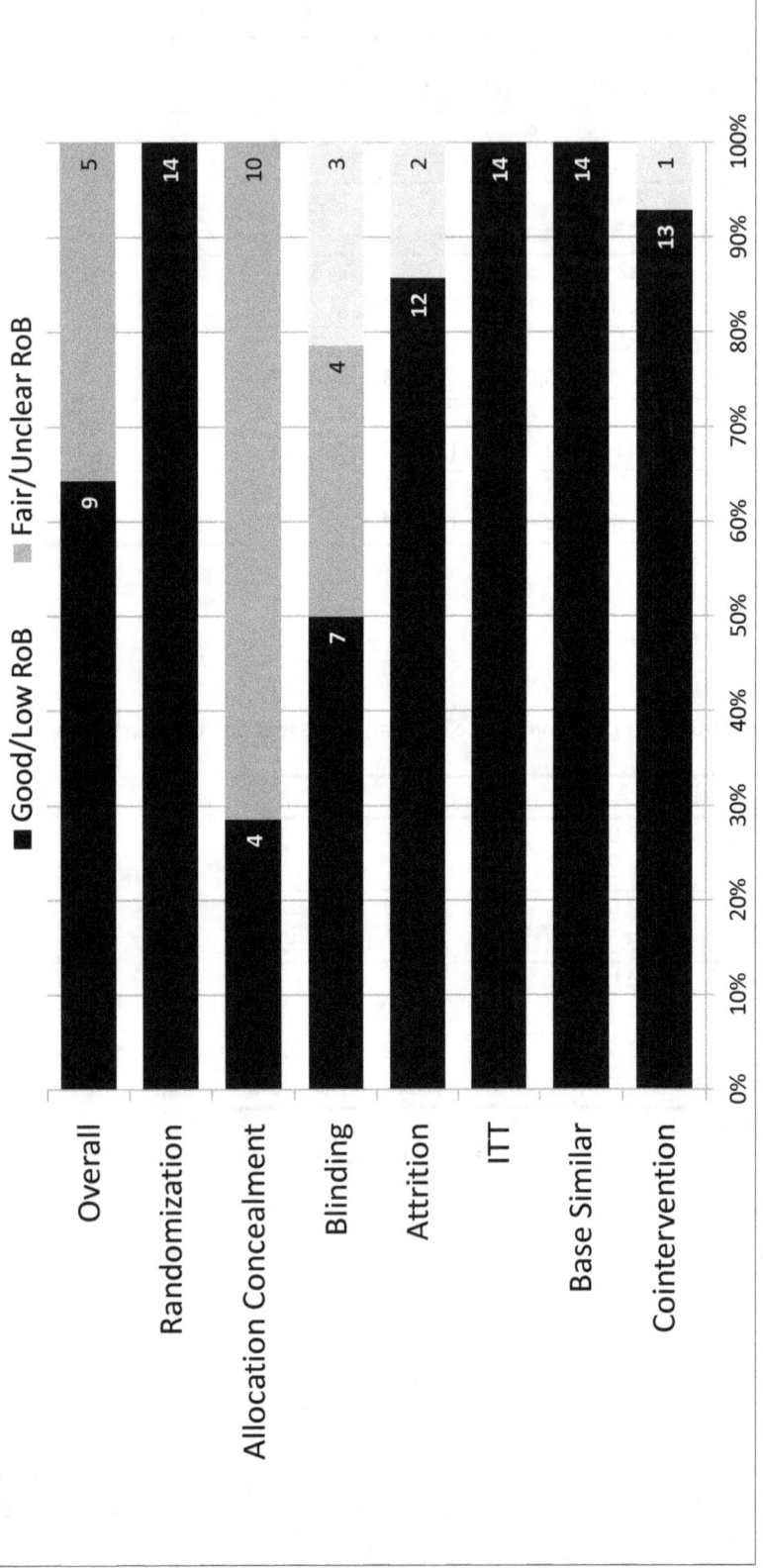

The numbers within the bars represent the number of studies within each category.

Overall: Good, fair, or poor quality study

Randomization: What is the risk of selection bias (biased allocation to interventions) due to inadequate generation of a randomized sequence?

Allocation Concealment: What is the risk of selection bias (biased allocation to interventions) due to inadequate concealment of allocations before assignment?

Blinding: Outcome Assessor Blinding—or each main outcome or class of outcomes, what was the risk of detection bias due to knowledge of the allocated interventions by outcome assessment (lack of outcome assessor blinding)?

Attrition: For each main outcome or class of outcomes, what is the risk of attrition bias due to amount, nature, or handling of incomplete outcome data?

ITT: Intention-to-Treat—Were all randomized participants analyzed in the group to which they were allocated?

Base Similar: Groups Similarity—Were the groups similar at baseline regarding the most important prognostic indicators?

Cointervention: Were co-interventions avoided or similar?

34

Figure 4. Random effects model meta-analysis of ICD vs. no ICD for all-cause mortality

Study	Comparator	Max f/up	Mean f/up*	HR (95% CI)		ICD	No ICD n/N	Quality
COMPANION (Bristow 2004) A	CRT-D v No ICD	1000 d	~1.3 y	0.64 [0.48, 0.85]		105/595	77/308	Fair
COMPANION (Bristow 2004) B†	CRT-D v CRT-P†	1000 d	~1.3 y	0.81 [0.63, 1.05]††		105/595†	131/617†	Fair
MADIT II (Moss 2002)§	No ICD	4 y	1.7 y	0.69 [0.51, 0.93]		105/742	97/490	Good
AMIOVIRT (Strickberger 2003)	Amiodarone	52 mo	~2.0 y	0.87 [0.29, 2.58]‡		6/51	7/52	Good
MADIT (Moss 1996)	No ICD	5 y	2.3 y	0.46 [0.26, 0.82]		15/95	39/101	Fair
DEFINITE (Kadish 2004)	No ICD	5 y	2.4 y	0.65 [0.40, 1.06]		28/229	40/229	Fair
DINAMIT (Hohnloser 2004)	No ICD	4 y	2.5 y	1.08 [0.76, 1.54]		62/332	58/342	Good
CABG-Patch (Bigger 1997)	No ICD	4 y	2.7 y	1.03 [0.75, 1.41]		101/446	95/454	Fair
IRIS (Steinbeck 2009)	No ICD	6 y	3.1 y	1.04 [0.81, 1.34]		116/445	117/453	Good
SCD-HeFT (Bardy 2005) A	No ICD	5 y	3.8 y]	0.77 [0.62, 0.96]		182/829	244/847	Good
SCD-HeFT (Bardy 2005) B†	Amiodarone†	5 y	3.8 y]	0.74 [0.61, 0.90]††		182/829†	240/845†	Fair¶
CAT (Bänsch 2002)	No ICD	7 y	5.5 y	0.71 [0.34, 1.46]‡		13/50	17/54	Good
Summary estimate (n=7)				0.69 [0.60, 0.79]	P<0.001	i²=0%		
(with CABG-Patch; n=8)				0.73 [0.62, 0.87]	P<0.001	i²=36%		
(with IRIS, DINAMIT; n=9)				0.76 [0.65, 0.91]	P=0.002	i²=44%		
(with IRIS, DINAMIT, CABG-Patch; n=10)				0.80 [0.58, 0.94]	P=0.009	i²=51%		

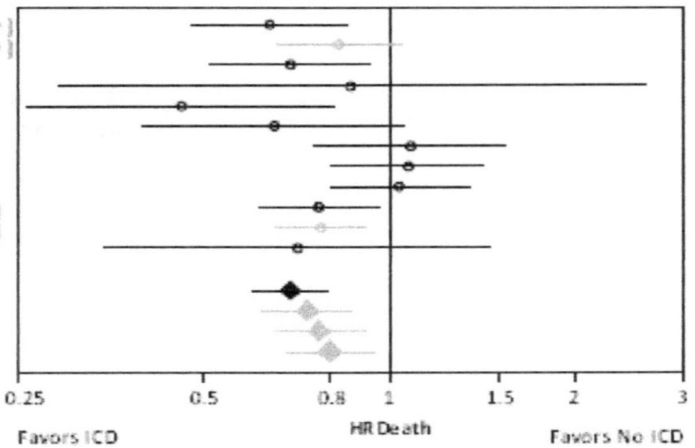

CI = confidence interval; CRT-D = cardiac resynchronization therapy with a defibrillator; CRT-P = cardiac resynchronization therapy with a pacemaker (without a defibrillator); f/up = followup; HR = hazard ratio; ICD = implantable cardiac defibrillator; n/N = total events (deaths)/total analyzed. See page 16 for study acronyms.

* Values in brackets are medians; ~ signifies approximate.
† Not included in meta-analyses (the alternative comparison for each study was the only comparison included in meta-analyses).
‡ Hazard ratio and confidence interval estimated from reported data.
§ The 8-year (maximum) followup of MADIT II (Barsheshet 2011) excluded because it analyzed an arbitrary subgroup of ICD group only.
¶ Differential use of beta blockers between ICD and amiodarone groups (but not between ICD and no ICD groups).

Figure 5. Differences in cumulative death proportions between ICD and no ICD, by year

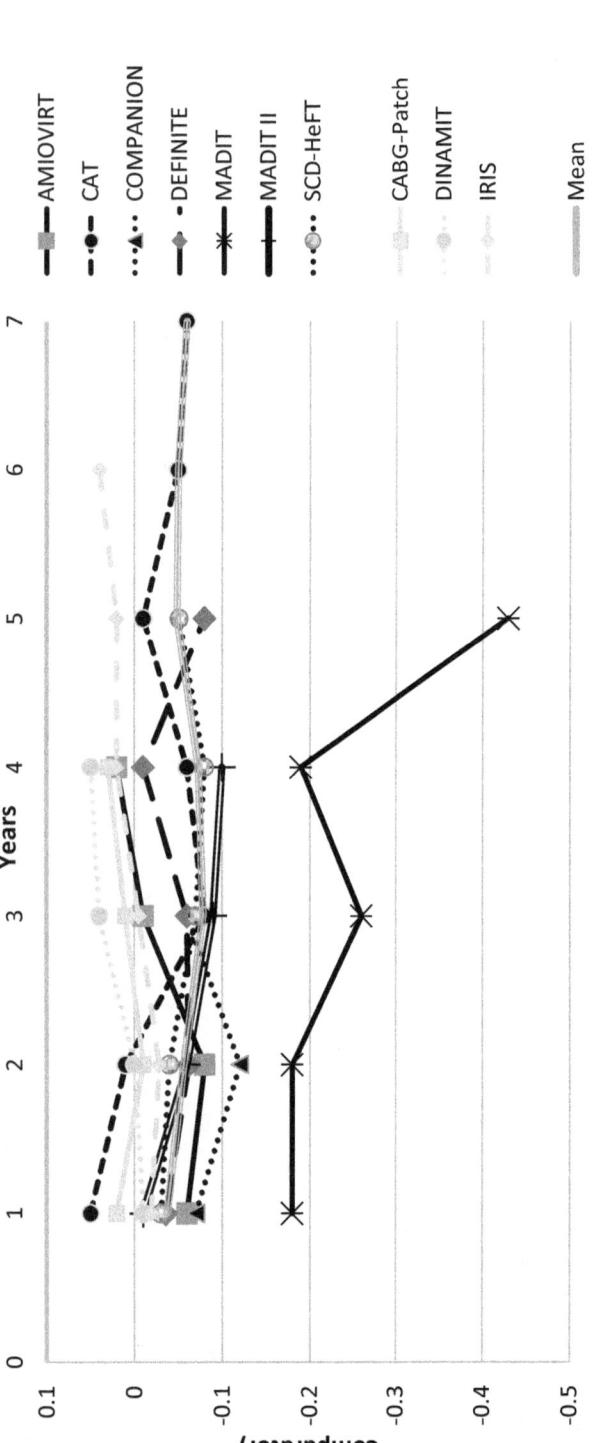

Study	No. at Risk							Total Deaths (Proportion) ICD	Comparator	Mean Followup
		1	2	3	4	5	6			
AMIOVIRT	103	nd	nd	nd	nd			6 (0.11)	7 (0.13)	~2.0 y
CAT	104	98	96	89	81	67	49	13 (0.26)	17 (0.31)	5.5 y
COMPANION	903*	606†	205‡	3§				105 (0.17)	77 (0.25)	~15 mo (median)
DEFINITE	458	428	271	144	73	nd		28 (0.12)	40 (0.17)	29 mo
MADIT	196	147	101	60	34	3		15 (0.15)	39 (0.38)	27 mo
MADIT II	1232	832	444	175	12			105 (0.14)	97 (0.19)	20 mo
SCD-HeFT	1674	1560	1448	985	584	200		182 (0.21)	240 (0.28)	46 mo (median)
CABG-Patch	900	783	621	412	138			101 (0.22)	95 (0.2)	32 mo
DINAMIT	674	504	428	247	56			62 (0.19)	58 (0.18)	30 mo
IRIS	898	746	610	437	288	157		116 (0.26)	117 (0.25)	37 mo

ICD = implanted cardiac defibrillator, mo = months, y = years. See page 16 for study acronyms.
Data derived from digitized Kaplan-Meier curves. The mean difference curve is a rough average, weighted by number at risk or its imputed estimate, of studies excluding CABG-Patch, DINAMIT, and IRIS.

36

Figure 6. Random effects model meta-analysis of relative odds ratio of ICD vs. no ICD for arrhythmic death between women and men

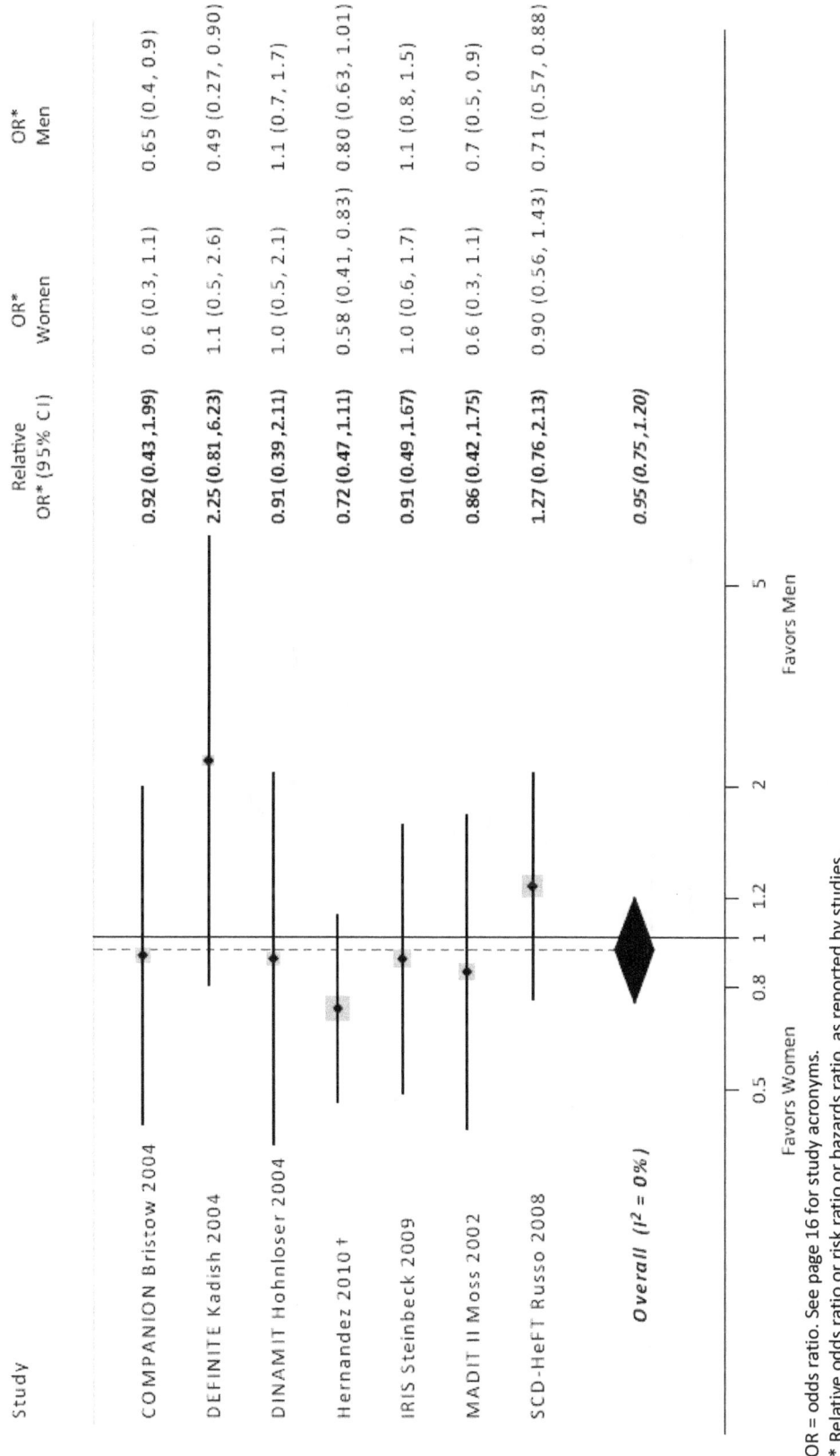

Study	Relative OR* (95% CI)	OR* Women	OR* Men
COMPANION Bristow 2004	0.92 (0.43 ,1.99)	0.6 (0.3 , 1.1)	0.65 (0.4, 0.9)
DEFINITE Kadish 2004	2.25 (0.81,6.23)	1.1 (0.5 , 2.6)	0.49 (0.27, 0.90)
DINAMIT Hohnloser 2004	0.91 (0.39 ,2.11)	1.0 (0.5 , 2.1)	1.1 (0.7, 1.7)
Hernandez 2010 †	0.72 (0.47 ,1.11)	0.58 (0.41 , 0.83)	0.80 (0.63 , 1.01)
IRIS Steinbeck 2009	0.91 (0.49 ,1.67)	1.0 (0.6 , 1.7)	1.1 (0.8 , 1.5)
MADIT II Moss 2002	0.86 (0.42 ,1.75)	0.6 (0.3 , 1.1)	0.7 (0.5 , 0.9)
SCD-HeFT Russo 2008	1.27 (0.76 ,2.13)	0.90 (0.56 , 1.43)	0.71 (0.57, 0.88)
Overall (I² = 0%)	0.95 (0.75 ,1.20)		

Favors Women   Favors Men

0.5   0.8   1   1.2   2   5

OR = odds ratio. See page 16 for study acronyms.
* Relative odds ratio or risk ratio or hazards ratio, as reported by studies.
† OPTIMIZE-HF and GWTG-H

37

Figure 7. Random effects model meta-analysis of relative odds ratio of ICD vs. no ICD for arrhythmic death between younger and older subgroups

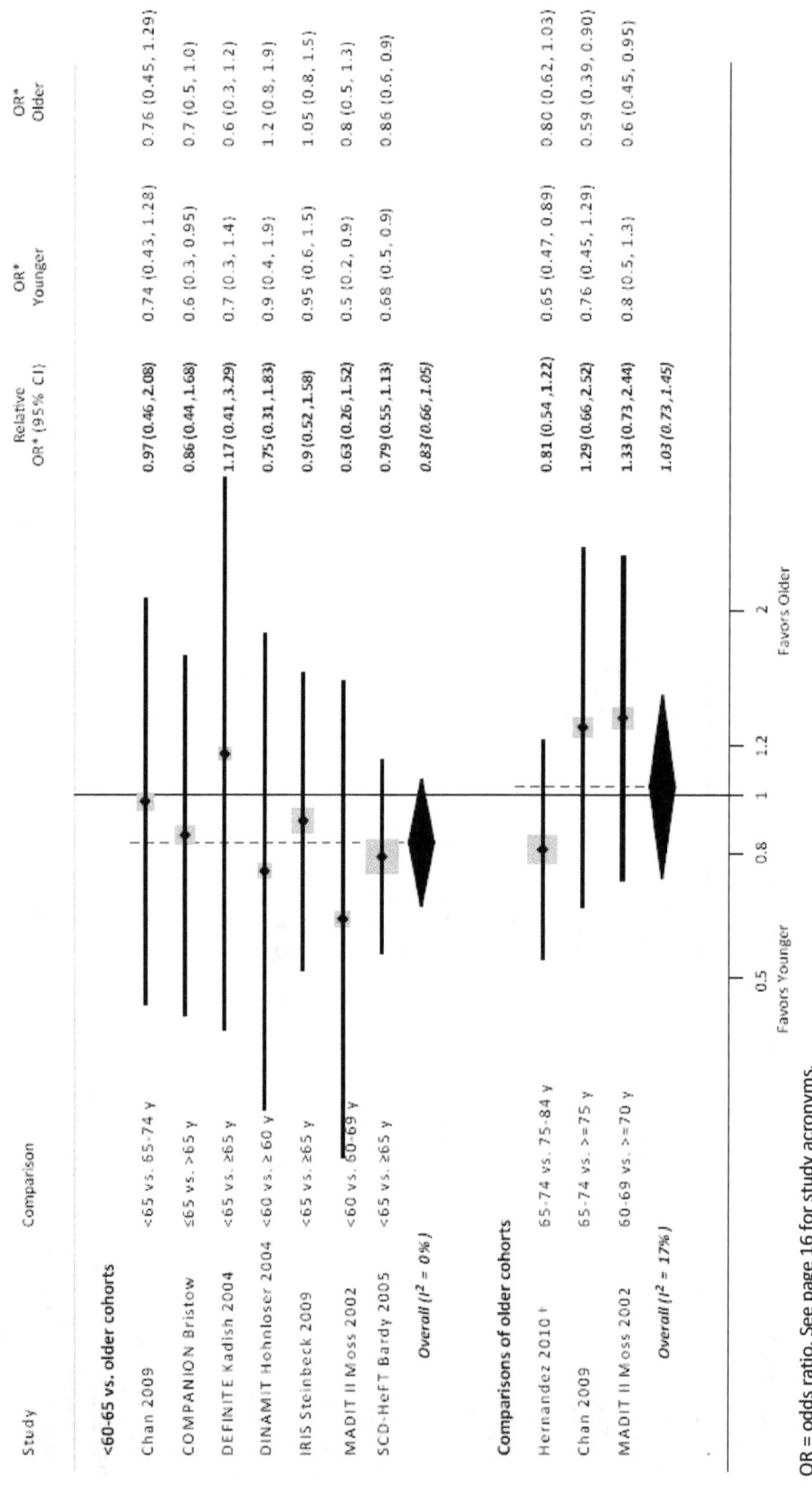

Study	Comparison	Relative OR* (95% CI)	OR* Younger	OR* Older
<60-65 vs. older cohorts				
Chan 2009	<65 vs. 65-74 y	0.97 (0.46, 2.08)	0.74 (0.43, 1.28)	0.76 (0.45, 1.29)
COMPANION Bristow	≤65 vs. >65 y	0.86 (0.44, 1.68)	0.6 (0.3, 0.95)	0.7 (0.5, 1.0)
DEFINITE Kadish 2004	<65 vs. ≥65 y	1.17 (0.41, 3.29)	0.7 (0.3, 1.4)	0.6 (0.3, 1.2)
DINAMIT Hohnloser 2004	<60 vs. ≥60 y	0.75 (0.31, 1.83)	0.9 (0.4, 1.9)	1.2 (0.8, 1.9)
IRIS Steinbeck 2009	<65 vs. ≥65 y	0.9 (0.52, 1.58)	0.95 (0.6, 1.5)	1.05 (0.8, 1.5)
MADIT II Moss 2002	<60 vs. 60-69 y	0.63 (0.26, 1.52)	0.5 (0.2, 0.9)	0.8 (0.5, 1.3)
SCD-HeFT Bardy 2005	<65 vs. ≥65 y	0.79 (0.55, 1.13)	0.68 (0.5, 0.9)	0.86 (0.6, 0.9)
Overall (I² = 0%)		0.83 (0.66, 1.05)		
Comparisons of older cohorts				
Hernandez 2010 †	65-74 vs. 75-84 y	0.81 (0.54, 1.22)	0.65 (0.47, 0.89)	0.80 (0.62, 1.03)
Chan 2009	65-74 vs. >=75 y	1.29 (0.66, 2.52)	0.76 (0.45, 1.29)	0.59 (0.39, 0.90)
MADIT II Moss 2002	60-69 vs. >=70 y	1.33 (0.73, 2.44)	0.8 (0.5, 1.3)	0.6 (0.45, 0.95)
Overall (I² = 17%)		1.03 (0.73, 1.45)		

OR = odds ratio. See page 16 for study acronyms.

* Relative odds ratio or risk ratio or hazards ratio, as reported by studies.

† OPTIMIZE-HF and GWTG-H

38

Figure 8. Random effects model meta-analysis of ICD vs. no ICD for arrhythmic death

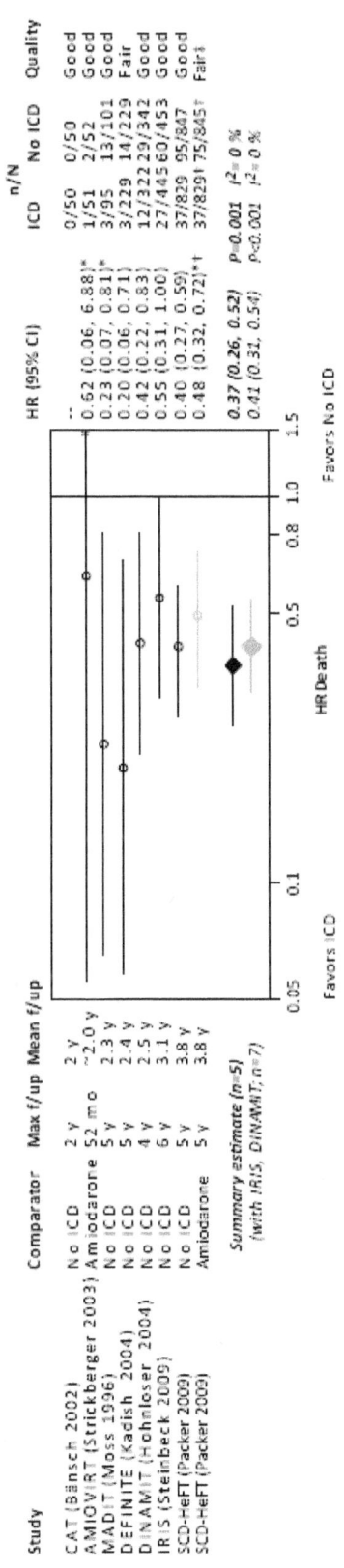

Study	Comparator	Max f/up	Mean f/up	HR (95% CI)	n/N ICD	No ICD	Quality
CAT (Bänsch 2002)	No ICD	2 y	2 y	--	0/50	0/50	Good
AMIOVIRT (Strickberger 2003)	Amiodarone	52 mo	~2.0 y	0.62 (0.06, 6.88)*	1/51	2/52	Good
MADIT (Moss 1996)	No ICD	5 y	2.3 y	0.23 (0.07, 0.81)*	3/95	13/101	Good
DEFINITE (Kadish 2004)	No ICD	5 y	2.4 y	0.20 (0.06, 0.71)	3/229	14/229	Fair
DINAMIT (Hohnloser 2004)	No ICD	4 y	2.5 y	0.42 (0.22, 0.83)	12/332	29/342	Good
IRIS (Steinbeck 2009)	No ICD	6 y	3.1 y	0.55 (0.31, 1.00)	27/445	60/453	Good
SCD-HeFT (Packer 2009)	No ICD	5 y	3.8 y	0.40 (0.27, 0.59)	37/829	95/847	Good
SCD-HeFT (Packer 2009)	Amiodarone	5 y	3.8 y	0.48 (0.32, 0.72)*†	37/829†	75/845†	Fair†

Summary estimate (n=5) 0.37 (0.26, 0.52) P=0.001 I^2= 0 %
(with IRIS, DINAMIT, n=7) 0.41 (0.31, 0.54) p<0.001 I^2= 0 %

HR Death — Favors ICD / Favors No ICD

~ = approximately; CI = confidence interval; f/up = followup; HR = hazard ratio; ICD = implantable cardiac defibrillator; n/N = total events (deaths)/total analyzed. See page 16 for study acronyms.

* Hazard ratio and confidence interval estimated from reported data.
† Not included in meta-analyses (the alternative comparison for each study was the only comparison included in meta-analyses).
‡ Differential use of beta blockers between ICD and amiodarone groups (but not between ICD and no ICD groups).

Figure 9. Differences in cumulative sudden cardiac/arrhythmia death proportions between ICD and no ICD, by year

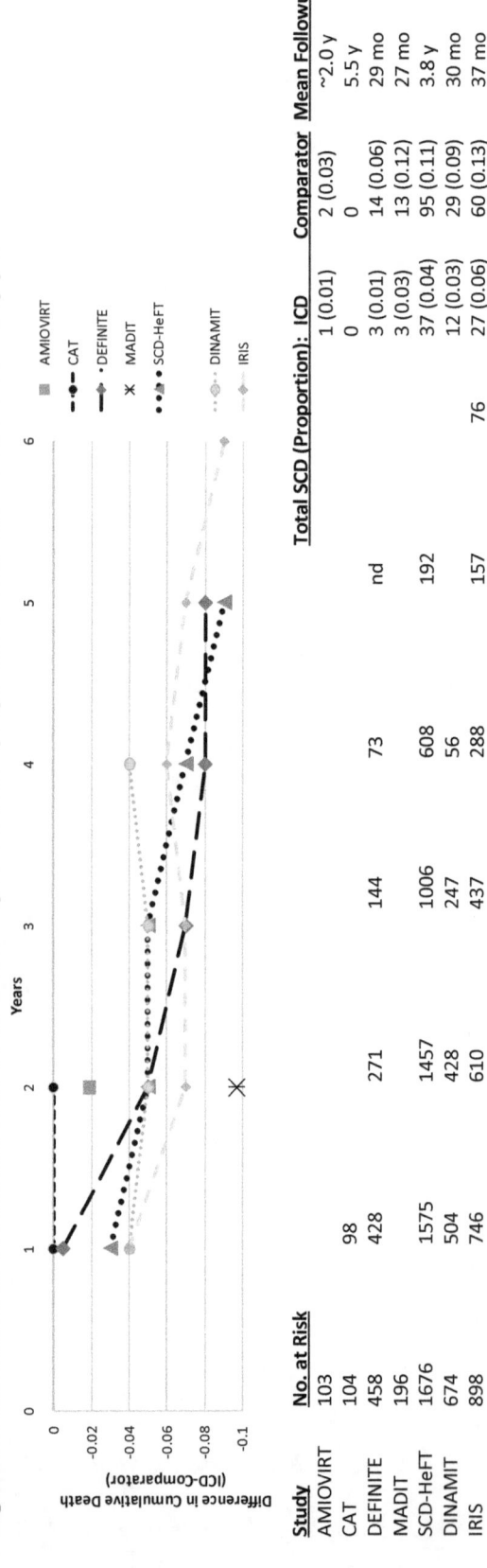

Study	No. at Risk					Total SCD (Proportion): ICD	Comparator	Mean Followup
AMIOVIRT	103					1 (0.01)	2 (0.03)	~2.0 y
CAT	104	98				0	0	5.5 y
DEFINITE	458	428	271	144		3 (0.01)	14 (0.06)	29 mo
MADIT	196			73	nd	3 (0.03)	13 (0.12)	27 mo
SCD-HeFT	1676	1575	1457	1006	608	192	37 (0.04)	95 (0.11)	3.8 y
DINAMIT	674	504	428	247	56	12 (0.03)	29 (0.09)	30 mo
IRIS	898	746	610	437	288	157	27 (0.06)	60 (0.13)	37 mo

ICD = implanted cardiac defibrillator, mo = months, SCD = sudden cardiac death, y = years. See page 16 for study acronyms.
Data derived from digitized Kaplan-Meier curves, where available. AMIOVIRT, CAT, and MADIT did not report Kaplan Meier curves. CAT reported data for years 1 and 2. AMIOVIRT and MADIT reported only total numbers of death; the points for these two studies are plotted at their approximate mean duration of followup.

40

Key Questions 1b & 1c:
In Candidates for ICD Implantation for Primary Prevention of SCD, What Are the Effects of ICD with ATP versus ICD alone, or of ICD with CRT versus ICD alone on Clinical Outcomes and Patient-Reported Outcomes?
How Do Outcomes Vary Within Subgroups?

We searched for studies that examined the effect of ATP added to ICD, or the effect of CRT added to ICD, versus ICD alone. We did not include comparisons of shock algorithms or algorithms pertaining to pacing for bradycardia, different manufacturers of equivalent ICDs, or different numbers of leads used *per se* (except as required for CRT). The findings and strength of evidence for outcomes with sufficient evidence for the comparison of CRT-D versus ICD are summarized in **Table 8**.

No study examined the effect of adding ATP in patients undergoing ICD implantation for predominantly primary prevention. Four studies that met eligibility criteria directly compared ICD with CRT versus ICD alone (**Table 10**).[73,111,112] All focused on congestive heart failure outcomes, which were not outcomes of interest for this review. We did not meta-analyze the studies since there were only two sufficiently large studies to analyze death and meta-analysis would not provide a better estimate of the effect size than evaluating the two large trials separately.

Table 10. Summary of findings for CRT-D vs. ICD

Outcome	Study Design: No. Studies (N)	Findings	Strength of Evidence
All-cause mortality	CRT-D vs. ICD RCT: 4 (3,743)	• The 2 larger trials found either no difference (HR = 1.00) or a significant benefit with CRT-D (HR = 0.75). No differences in effect were found between patients with ischemic or nonischemic heart disease or with NYHA Class II or III cardiomyopathy • There was no evidence regarding the comparison of CRT-D and ICD in subgroups of patients or based on different characteristics of facilities where ICDs are implanted.	Insufficient

Abbreviations: CI = confidence interval, CRT-D = cardiac resynchronization therapy-defibrillator, HR = hazard ratio, ICD = implantable cardioverter–defibrillator, No. = number, NYHA = New York Heart Association, RCT = randomized, controlled trial

Studies

MADIT-CRT

MADIT-CRT[73] compared the combination of CRT plus ICD (CRT-D) with ICD alone in patients with ischemic or nonischemic cardiomyopathy, an LVEF <30 percent, and QRS duration >130 ms. We assessed the study to be of good quality. Patients' mean age was 64 years and three-quarters of them were men. Their mean LVEF was 24 percent. About 15 percent of patients had NYHA Class I ischemic heart disease, 40 percent had Class II ischemic heart disease, and 45 percent had Class II nonischemic heart disease. This distribution reflects the study's eligibility criteria. About 65 percent had a QRS duration≥150 ms. About 30 percent had diabetes.

After 5 years of followup, 74 of 1089 patients (6.8%) who received CRT-D died and 53 of 731 (7.3%) patients with ICD only died. The HR for all-cause death with CRT-D versus ICD only was 1.00 (95% CI 0.69, 1.44). The effects of adding CRT in either patients with ischemic or with nonischemic cardiomyopathy were similar and not statistically significantly different between populations. For patients with ischemic heart disease (NYHA Class I or II), the HR was 1.06 (95% CI 0.68, 1.64); for patients with nonischemic heart disease (NYHA Class II only), the HR was 0.87 (95% CI 0.44, 1.70). MADIT-CRT did not evaluate other outcomes of interest to this review or other subgroups of interest for all-cause mortality.

In a comparison of patients who had and who did not have coronary revascularization prior to ICD placement,[113] the frequency of combined ventricular tachyarrhythmia or death did not differ among patients with CRT-D or ICD, regardless of coronary revascularization history or time since coronary revascularization.

RAFT

RAFT compared CRT-D with ICD alone in patients with NYHA Class II or III heart failure, LVEF≤30 percent, QRS duration ≥200 msec, sinus rhythm or controlled atrial fibrillation, and planned ICD implantation.[74] The study was not restricted to patients receiving ICDs for primary prevention, but only 14 percent had a history of a prior SCD episode. We assessed the study to be of good quality. Patients' mean age was 66 years and 83 percent were men. Their mean LVEF was 23 percent and 80 percent had NYHA Class II heart failure; the remainder had Class III heart failure. Their mean QRS duration was 158 ms. About one-third had diabetes.

During a total of 6 years of followup (mean 40 months), 236 of 904 (26%) patients who had received ICD alone died and 186 of 894 (21%) with CRT-D died; thus the HR for all-cause death was 0.75 (95% CI 0.64, 0.87), favoring CRT-D. No difference in effect size was found for patients with Class II or Class II heart failure. The HR for all-cause death among those with Class II heart failure was 0.71 (0.56, 0.91) and for those with Class III heart failure 0.79 (0.58, 1.08).

Diab 2011

In the only RCT of ICD for primary prevention without an acronym name, Diab 2011 compared CRT-D with ICD alone in patients with NYHA Class III or IV heart failure, LVEF <35 percent, and QRS duration ≥120 ms, but with echocardiographic evidence of no mechanical dyssynchrony.[112] We assessed the study to be of good quality, although underpowered for clinical outcomes. Patients' mean age was 66 years and 89 percent were men. Their mean LVEF was 26 percent. Almost 90 percent had NYHA Class III heart failure. Their mean QRS duration was 138 ms. The percentage of patients with diabetes was not reported.

After 6 months of followup, 2 of 22 (9%) patients who received ICD alone died, but none of 24 patients with CRT-D died. One patient in each group was hospitalized for surgical lead implantation or repositioning. No other outcomes of interest and no subgroup analyses were reported.

MENDMI

MENDMI compared CRT-D with ICD alone in patients with a recent MI (within 3 to 16 days), LVEF ≤35 percent, and a wall motion abnormality on echocardiogram in >5 of 16 cardiac segments.[111] Based on their recent MIs, current guidelines would not recommend ICD in these patients. We assessed the study to be of fair quality, having differential attrition rates. It was also underpowered for clinical outcomes. Patients' mean age was 57 years and 75 percent were men. Their mean LVEF was 28 percent. About two-thirds had NYHA Class II or III heart failure. Their mean QRS duration was 88 ms. Before a protocol revision, diabetes had been an exclusion criterion, so only 8 percent of patients had diabetes.

In the trial, 42 patients received CRT-D and 38 received ICD alone. Within 1 year of followup, one patient died in each arm. The only hospitalization postimplantation occurred after a failed ICD induction, but it was not reported which ICD the patient had.

Summary

Four RCTs compared CRT-D with ICD alone, one of which included patients with very recent MIs (within 2 weeks) (**Table 11**). The two large trials had discordant findings, such that MADIT-CRT found no difference in death between CRT-D and ICD alone in patients with ischemic NYHA Class I cardiomyopathy or ischemic or nonischemic NYHA Class II cardiomyopathy, while RAFT found a statistically significant 25 percent reduction in death with CRT-D in patients with Class II or III ischemic or nonischemic cardiomyopathy. The other two RCTs were greatly underpowered for clinical outcomes and therefore adds little to the evidence base for outcomes of interest to this review. The evidence is insufficient to determine whether there is a difference in death between CRT and ICD alone for primary prevention or whether there may be a subpopulation of patients (captured by RAFT) who may benefit from CRT-D (**Table 8**). Both large trials found no difference in effect between either patients with ischemic or nonischemic heart disease or patients with Class II or III cardiomyopathy. There is insufficient evidence for all other outcomes and comparisons of interest, including differential effects of CRT-D and ICD on all-cause mortality for other populations of patients or different characteristics of facilities where ICDs are implanted; the effect of CRT-D versus ICD on SCD, sustained ventricular tachyarrhythmia, general QoL, or other general patient-reported outcomes. No study examined the effect of adding ATP in patients undergoing ICD implantation for predominantly primary prevention.

Table 11. ICD vs. CRT-D: Study characteristics

Study Author Year PMID	Intervention (Control)	NYHA class	Ischemic	Non-ischemic	Non sustained VT	% LVEF	Total N	Primary outcome	Duration followup	ICD type/No. of leads	Enrollment period
Diab 2011 21700757	ICD (CRT-D)	III, IV	Yes	Yes	nd	≤35	73	Peak oxygen consumption	6 mo	nd	2007-2009
MADIT-CRT Moss 2009 19723701	ICD (CRT-D)	I, II	Yes	Yes	No	≤30	1820	All-cause death or nonfatal heart failure event	4 y mean 2.4 y	Single-, dual-chamber vs. biventricular	12/22/2004-4/23/2008
MENDMI Chung 2010 20852059	ICD (CRT-D)	I, II, III	nd	Yes	NR	≤35	80	Change in LV end-diastolic volume at 12 mo	12 mo	Single-, dual-chamber vs. biventricular	2005-2008
RAFT Tang, 2010 21073365	ICD (CRT-D)	II, III	Yes	Yes	nd	≤30	1798*	Death or hospitalization for heart failure	40 mo mean 3.3 y	nd	1/2003-2/2009

CRT-D = cardiac resynchronization therapy defibrillator, ICD = implantable cardiac defibrillator, LV = left ventricular, MADIT-CRT = Multicenter Automatic Defibrillator Implantation Trial with Cardiac Resynchronization Therapy, MENDMI = Prevention of Myocardial Enlargement and Dilation Post Myocardial Infarction Study, mo = month, nd = not documented, NYHA = New York Heart Association, VT = ventricular tachycardia, y = year

* 20% of patients had ICDs implanted for secondary prevention of sudden cardiac death.

44

Table 11. CRT-D vs. ICD for primary prevention of SCD: Strength of evidence domains

Outcome	Study Design: No. Studies (N)	Study Limitations	Directness	Consistency	Precision	Reporting Bias	Other Issues	Finding and Strength of Evidence
All-cause mortality (≥1 y)	RCT: 4 (3,743)	Low RoB (3 good, 1 fair)	Direct	Inconsistent	Precise	Undetected		Insufficient The 2 larger trials found either no difference (HR = 1.00) or a significant benefit with CRT-D (HR = 0.75) No differences in effect were found between patients with ischemic or nonischemic heart disease or with NYHA Class II or III cardiomyopathy
All-cause mortality (30 d)	0							Insufficient
Sudden cardiac death (arrhythmic death)	0							Insufficient
Sustained ventricular tachyarrhythmia	0							Insufficient
Quality of life	0							Insufficient
Other patient-reported outcomes	RCT: 1 (46)	Low RoB (1 good)	Direct	Consistent	Imprecise	Undetected		Insufficient Unclear whether rates of hospitalization for surgical lead implantation or repositioning differ

CI = confidence interval, CRT-D = cardiac resynchronization therapy with defibrillator, HR = summary hazard ratio, ICD = implanted cardiac defibrillator, nRCS = nonrandomized comparative study, NYHA = New York Heart Association, RoB = risk of bias, RCT = randomized controlled trial.

Key Question 2a: What are the adverse events related to treatment with an ICD for primary prevention of SCD?

Key Question 2b: How do adverse events vary within subgroups?

Although this report is focused on primary prevention, for our review of adverse events, we also included studies of mixed populations of patients with ICDs for either primary or secondary prevention. This was done not only to enrich the evidence base but also because many adverse events are related to ICD placement rather than the indication for the device and thus are likely to be more similar than different across populations with primary and secondary indications.

We identified a total of 59 articles contributing data on adverse events, 14 with results for early adverse events, i.e. adverse events occurring during hospitalization for ICD implantation or up to 30 days after implantation, 33 studies contributing data for late adverse events and 22 studies on inappropriate shock. The findings and strength of evidence for adverse events related to ICD are summarized in **Table 12**.

Table 12. Summary of findings regarding adverse event

Outcome	Study Design: No. Studies (N)	Findings	Strength of Evidence
Early AEs (In-hospital)	RCT: 3 (3,867) Observational: 11 (356,515*) [overlapping cohorts]	During hospitalization, 2.8–3.6% of patients had any adverse event. Serious adverse events occurred in 1.2–1.35% after ICD placement. The most common specific adverse events were lead dislodgement (0.7–1.2%) and hematoma (0.8–1.1%). Other in-hospital adverse events occurred in ≤0.5% of patients receiving ICDs Based on within-study subgroups analyses, there may be higher rates of adverse events among patients receiving dual-chamber ICDs, CRT-D, among older patients, women, and those with ESRD. Physicians and hospitals with lower volume of implantation and operators other than electrophysiologists may have more adverse events.	High
Late AEs (Out of hospital)	RCT: 3 (2,149) Observational: 28 reports of 22 independent cohorts (99,725†)	Device-related adverse events occurred in <0.1–6.4% of ICD patients during 2–49 month followup. Other relatively common adverse events included lead malfunction (<0.1–3.9% during 1.5–40 month followup), infection (0.2–3.7% for 1.5–49 month followup), and thrombosis (0.2–2.9% for 1.5–49 month followup). Based on within-study subgroup analyses, there may be more lead-related adverse events in women. There was no apparent difference in adverse events between CRT-D and ICD or between dual and single chamber ICDs.	Low
Inappropriate shock	RCT: 1 (249) Observational: 21 reports of 17 independent cohorts (212,063‡)	Inappropriate shock occurred in 3–21% of patients during 1–5 year followup. Based on within-study subgroup analyses, there may be more inappropriate shocks among younger patients Evidence on the difference in inappropriate shocks between dual and single chamber ICDs was inconsistent. Limited data show no apparent difference in inappropriate shocks between CRT-D and ICD.	Moderate

Abbreviations: AE = adverse event, CRT-D = cardiac resynchronization therapy-defibrillator, ESRD = end stage renal disease, ICD = implantable cardioverter–defibrillator, No. =number, RCT = randomized, controlled trial

* Largest independent N

† Largest independent N. Two large cohorts: N=38,992 (PMID 21795298), N=15,387 (PMID 19925609)

† Largest independent N. One large cohort: N=185,778 (PMID 21098452)

Figure 10 and **Appendix Table 11** shows the quality of reporting for harms across the comparative and cohort studies according to the questions shown in the legend. All reports from one database (i.e., the NCDR ICD Database and the EPD-Vision Database) were graded jointly. Most studies prespecified at least one adverse event in the Methods section, and many used a standardized or precise definition. It seemed that all prespecified harms were reported. Most studies reported the active collection of harms, although some did not comment on ascertainment. Very few studies explicitly stated whether passive (patient-initiated) ascertainment was used (as either the primary or supplementary mode of collection). Most studies described the timing of adverse event collection at regularly scheduled postimplantation visits. Our review only included studies providing the number of patients experiencing harms (numerator) and the total number at risk (denominator).

Overall, our screening and selection criteria enriched the database for studies with purposeful reporting of adverse events. The strength of evidence for early (in-hospital) adverse events is high as they are derived from a registry with standard definitions, wide capture, and a large number of patients. The strength of evidence for late adverse events is low because there are only a few studies for each outcome and outcome definitions and ascertainment varied. The strength of evidence for inappropriate shocks was moderate with good data ascertainment but imprecise rates across studies.

Early Adverse Events from the NCDR ICD Registry

We identified 11 studies reporting harms ascertained in the NCDR ICD registry (**Appendix Table 12**).[62,66,67,114-121] These studies ranged in size from 44,805 to 356,515 patients; the patients overlapped to a large degree across studies; therefore the patient populations are not independent. The percentage of patients receiving an ICD for primary prevention in the individual studies ranged from 68 to 100 percent (with one study not reporting the proportion). Although the NCDR ICD registry is a comprehensive database with purposeful data collection, it is restricted to the data capture during the hospitalization for ICD implantation and may not capture all early adverse events.

Appendix Table 13 shows the range of rates for each adverse event category across the 10 reports reporting rates.[62,66,67,114-118,120,121] One additional study provided subgroup data only.[119] **Table 13** presents a summary of the early adverse event rates across studies. The percentage of patients with any adverse events ranged from 2.77 to 3.55 percent across cohorts. Wei 2011[121] reported a substantially higher adverse event percentage (4.6%) than other studies, so we did not include it in the range. The higher rates of adverse events in Wei 2011 most likely occurred because the study involved patients who were at higher risk; namely, it included patients who had a B-type natriuretic peptide value at baseline, a laboratory test that which is tested in patients evaluated for heart failure. This study also did not focus on patients with a first ICD.

The most commonly reported specific early adverse events were lead dislodgement (0.73-1.2% of patients) and hematoma (0.84-1.1% of patients). All other specific adverse events occurred in less than 0.51 percent of patients.

Subgroup Analyses

All 11 studies using the NCDR ICD database reported subgroup analyses (**Appendix Table 14**). Statistical tests were not always provided for comparison of adverse event rates in subgroups, but 7 of the 11 studies reported statistical comparisons for at least one subgroup.

The rate of any adverse events was consistently and significantly higher in groups with dual-chamber ICDs and CRT-Ds (vs. single-chamber), older age, female sex, end-stage renal disease (ESRD), and implantation either by physicians or at hospitals with a low volume of implantations performed. The findings from analyses for specific adverse events were consistent with these subgroup effects or were not statistically significant. The only exception is a study showing a lower, rather than higher, risk of coronary venous dissection in patients with ESRD,[114] but the overall rate of this complication was low at 0.15 percent.

Other results of subgroup analyses were variable. Findings from two analyses (Tsai 2011 and Cheng 2010) for race and ethnicity were inconsistent.[62,120] Results for diabetes were non-significant in two studies. Haines 2011[117] found no statistically significant difference in the risk of an adverse event or death in patients who had received an ICD for primary prevention versus those who received an ICD for secondary prevention.

Four studies used the NCDR database to ascertain the rates of adverse events according to physician training.[62,66,67,120] In general, electrophysiologists had the lowest (or among the lowest) rates of adverse events. Tsai 2011[120] found a statistically higher odds ratio (OR) for any adverse event or death associated with surgeons (OR 1.49, P<0.001), nonelectrophysiologist cardiologists (OR 1.20, P<0.001), or other specialists (OR 1.18, P<0.05) rather than board-certified electrophysiologists. Cheng 2010[62] reported a higher risk of lead dislodgement in association with physicians trained under alternative pathways (HR 1.23; 95% CI 1.07, 1.45), and a trend for surgery board–certified physicians (HR 1.22; 95% CI 0.95, 1.56) as compared with electrophysiologists. Freeman 2012[67] reported the lowest rates of any adverse event for electrophysiologists but did not report statistical comparisons among physician groups. Finally, Curtis 2009[66] compared the rates of adverse events across electrophysiologists, nonelectrophysiologist cardiologists, thoracic surgeons, and other specialists. The percentages of any complication and of any major complication differed statistically significantly across the four groups, with the lowest percentages in the electrophysiologist group. Among common, specific adverse events, electrophysiologists had the lowest rates of hematoma, lead dislodgement, pneumothorax, and cardiac arrest. Other outcomes occurred in 0.1 percent or less of patients, with zero to five events in at least one subgroup; thus the estimates are not reliable.

Comparative Studies

There is limited comparative evidence on early adverse events for ICDs with different device features or numbers of leads (**Appendix Table 15 and Appendix Table 16**). MADIT-CRT[73] compared in-hospital and 30-day rates of adverse events in ICD and CRT-D recipients, which were as follows: coronary venous dissection with pericardial effusion (0% [ICD] vs. 0.5% [CRT-D]), pneumothorax (0.8 vs. 1.7%), infection (0.7 vs. 1.1%), and pocket hematoma requiring evacuation (2.5 vs. 3.3%). 30-day adverse events comparing ICD with CRT-D were also reported by RAFT: coronary sinus dissection (0 vs. 1.2%), hemothorax or pneumothorax (0.9 vs. 1.2%), pocket infection requiring intervention (1.8 vs. 2.4%), pocket hematoma requiring evacuation (1.2 vs. 1.6%) and lead dislodgement requiring revision (0.1 vs. 0.5%).[74] Neither study reported between-group statistical findings, but there was a trend toward higher percentages in the CRT-D arm than in the ICD arm.

ADRIA (A+ versus DR Clinical Investigation of Arrhythmia Discrimination)[122] compared in-hospital adverse events associated with receipt of a single-lead ICD with integrated atrial sensing rings versus a dual-chamber ICD. No statistical differences were found for pneumothorax (0.8% for both ICDs) or ventricular perforation (0 vs. 0.8%, respectively).

Late Adverse Events from Cohort Studies

We identified 28 studies of 500 or more patients that reported late adverse events occurring 30 or more days after ICD implantation (**Appendix Table 17**).[76,123-149] This includes ICD arms from MADIT II[76]) and SCD-Heft[145] as well as four studies derived from one database, the Leiden University Medical Center Cardiology Information System (EPD-Vision)[124,128,139,141] **Table 14** presents a summary of the late adverse event rates across studies.

In contrast with the studies in the NCDR ICD database, the literature overall had no standardization of outcome definitions across long-term studies. We tabulated device- and lead-related adverse events as they were reported (**Appendix Table 19**). Eight studies provided data on device-related events, namely malfunction requiring replacement or revision or dislocation.[127,130,132,134,139,140,142,146] The duration of followup was 2.6 to 70 months. The percentage of patients with malfunction or dislocation ranged from <0.1 to 6.4 percent.

One study reported that 6.1 percent of patients with recalled ICD devices experienced device-related adverse events with a 70 month followup.[146] (**Appendix Table 20**).

Sixteen studies provided data on lead-related adverse events, such as malfunction, failure, dislodgement, fracture, need for replacement, or revision or repositioning (**Appendix Table 20**).[76,124,125,127,129-132,135-137,140-143,149] The rates of these events ranged from <0.1 to 19 percent. Twelve studies reported rates from <0.1 to only 3.9 percent and had followup of 1.5 to 86 months. One study, by Morrison, reported reported a 4-year lead survival rate of 98.7 percent.[136] Four studies reported higher rates and had long followup periods (35 months, 43 months, 49 months and 8 years). Lead dysfunction was reported in 16.5 percent of patients at 35 months,[129] and lead revisions, in 19 percent at 43 months.[125] These two studies may have overlapping patient populations. High voltage lead defects were reported in 7.0 percent of patients with 49 month followup.[143] In addition, van Rees 2012, which reported 3.9 percent lead failure at 41 months, reported a cumulative 11.5 percent rate of lead failure at 8 years, the longest followup time reported for this outcome.[141]

Seven studies provided data on lead-related adverse events for the recalled Sprint Fidelis leads with followup ranging from 32 to 86 months (**Appendix Table 20**). Five of these studies reported a failure or a malfunction rate of between 7.1 and 8.4 percent.[123,126,131,144,147] The sixth study reported a 4-year lead survival rate of 87 percent,[136] which corresponds at most to a 13 percent failure rate. A *post hoc* analysis of patients in RAFT who received Sprint Fidelis leads reports 5.5 percent of patients had lead failure over 39 months and a lead fracture rate of 1.65 percent per year.[149]

Twelve studies provided data on infection, with followup periods of 1.5 to 49 months (**Appendix Table 21**).[76,124,127,128,130,132-134,138-141] The definition of infection varied across the studies, as did the severity and consequence of the observed cases. Additionally, it was not always possible to ascertain whether the infections reported in cohort studies included post-operative infection. Across all studies, the rate of infection ranged from 0.2 to 3.7 percent.

Four studies reported the rates of thrombosis (**Appendix Table 21**).[133,134,143,145] Among patients in SCD-HeFT without atrial fibrillation or flutter at baseline 2.9 percent experienced a thromboembolic event.[145] Three studies reported deep vein thrombosis rates of 0.2 to 1.0 percent with 1.5 to 49 month followup.[133,134,143]

Subgroup Analyses

We identified 12 articles that reported subgroup analyses of late (out of hospital) adverse events in ICD recipients (**Appendix Table 22**).[123,126,132,134,135,138,142,144,147,149-151] Of these, 11 studies reported statistical comparisons among subgroups for at least one outcome. Five studies compared rates of adverse events between patients receiving ICDs for primary prevention versus those with ICDs for secondary prevention.[123,132,142,144,147] No statistically significant differences were found between the two groups for surgical revision, lead dislodgement, recalled lead failure, or infection.

Four studies found statistically significantly higher rates of lead-related adverse events among women compared with men.[123,126,135,144] For other outcomes and subgroups, the evidence is sparse, with only one study addressing each subgroup comparison or two or more studies showing inconsistent findings.

Comparative Studies

There is limited comparative evidence on late (out of hospital) adverse events for ICDs with different device features or numbers of leads (**Appendix Table 15 and Appendix Table 16**). These studies have limited followup which may under-appreciate the rate of adverse events. Two RCTs report rates of late adverse events in ICD groups versus CRT-D groups.[73,111] MADIT-CRT reported the rates of total device-related adverse events as 5.2 vs. 4.5 per 100 device-months in ICD and CRT-D groups, respectively (without statistical comparison provided).[73] In the MENDMI study of 80 patients, after 1 year of followup, the composite adverse event was 42 percent with ICD and 52 percent with CRT-D (not statistically significant).[111] This prespecified composite outcome included LV lead dislodgement, postimplantation LV lead repositioning, permanent failure to deliver biventricular pacing, ventricular tachyarrhythmia, hospitalization due to cardiac causes and all-cause mortality.

ADRIA compared adverse events in patients who received a single-lead ICD with integrated atrial sensing rings to those with a dual-chamber ICD. At 1 year, ventricular lead–related adverse events were not statistically significantly different at 5.6 percent and 4.0 percent, respectively.[122]

Inappropriate Shock

We identified fifteen studies which provided data on inappropriate shocks in a cohort of at least 500 patients receiving ICDs.[51,125,129,130,135,136,152-160] Baseline information about these studies can be found in **Appendix Table 17**. The duration of followup ranged from 1 to 5 years. The percentage of patients experiencing inappropriate shocks was 3 to 21 percent overall (**Table 14, Appendix Table 18**). In four studies with 12 months of followup, percentages were 3 to 16 percent. For the other studies with 18 to 60 months followup, the percentage ranged from 8 to 21 percent. One study reported rates per year and found 2.4 percent of patients per year had inappropriate or unadjudicated shocks.[51] MADIT-RIT found that programming of ICD therapies for tachyarrhythmias of ≥ 200 beats per minute or with a prolonged delay in therapy at ≥ 170 beats per minute, as compared with conventional programming, was associated with reductions in inappropriate shock.[60]

Subgroup Analyses

We identified 13 articles that reported subgroup analyses of inappropriate shock in ICD recipients (**Appendix Table 22**).[93,125,129,135,148,150,151,153-155,159,161,162] All of these studies reported statistical comparisons for at least one subgroup comparison. Five studies compared rates of inappropriate shock between patients receiving ICDs for primary prevention versus those with ICDs for secondary prevention.[129,148,153,159,162] Only one of these found a statistically significant difference with fewer shocks in the primary prevention group.[153]

Five studies found lower rates of inappropriate shocks in older patients.[125,141,153,155,162] Age cut-offs varied between studies (more than 66.4 [the cohort mean age], 70, or 75 years, or per 10-year increase). In four of these, the difference was statistically significant. The fifth study did not report a statistical comparison. There was mixed data regarding the subgroup effect on inappropriate shock for single- vs. dual-chamber ICDs and for diabetes.

Comparative Studies

We identified one RCT and one nRCS that compare inappropriate shock in patients implanted with ICDs with different device features or numbers of leads (**Appendix Table 15 and Appendix Table 16**).[122,156] ALTITUDE (the acronym is undefined) reported a 5-year rate of inappropriate shock as 16 percent among ICD recipients and 17 percent among CRT-D recipients (no statistical comparison provided).[156] ADRIA (described above) reported rates of inappropriate shock as 5.6 percent in both single- and dual-chamber ICD groups.[122]

Summary

The rates of adverse events captured early in the NCDR ICD database range from 2.8 to 3.6 percent and the serious adverse event rates ranges from 1.2 to 1.35 percent (**Table 15**). The most common early adverse events are lead dislodgement (in 0.7 to 1.2 percent of patients) and hematoma (in 0.8-1.1 percent). Other early in-hospital adverse events occur in 0.5 percent of patients or less. The strength of evidence for early adverse events is high (**Table 12**).

Higher rates of early adverse events have been shown in the following subgroups: patients implanted with dual-chamber ICDs or CRT-Ds (vs. single-chamber ICDs); patients who are older, female, or have ESRD; patients implanted by physicians with a lower implantation volume or by nonelectrophysiologists; and patients implanted at hospitals with a lower implantation volume.

Regarding late adverse events which were captured usually after the initial hospitalization for implantation, the percentage of patients with device-related adverse events with variable definitions ranged from <0.1 to 6.4 percent for followup durations of 2 to 49 months. For lead-related adverse events (malfunction, failure, dislodgement, fracture, or need for replacement or revision, or repositioning) the rates ranged from <0.1 to 3.9 percent of patients with followup durations from 1.5 to 40 months, but studies with longer followup times (35 to 96 months) reported rates of 7.0 to 19 percent. Failure of the Sprint Fidelis lead was reported in approximately 6 to 8 percent of patients followed for up to 7 years. Infections, variably defined, were reported in 0.2 to 3.7 percent of patients with followup of 1.5 to 49 months. There are limited data on thrombosis in long-term followup:one study reported a rate of thromboemolic events of 2.9 percent, with a 46 month followup, and three studies reported deep vein thrombosis rates of 0.2 and 1 percent, with followup periods of 1.5 to 49 months. Given the limited number of studies for each outcome and the variable definitions and methods of ascertainment, the strength of evidence for late adverse events is low. Subgroup analyses show female sex to be associated with more lead-related adverse events.

The percentage of patients who experience at least one inappropriate shock ranged from 3 to 21 percent for followup between 1 and 5 years. The strength of evidence for inappropriate shocks was moderate with good data ascertainment but imprecision due to varying percentages across studies. Subgroup analyses show older age to be associated with fewer inappropriate shocks.

The data from five comparative studies for early and late adverse events and inappropriate shock fail to show differences across ICDs with different device features.

Table 14. Percentage of patients with early (in-hospital) adverse events in NCDR ICD database

Outcomes	No. Studies* (Largest N)	Adverse Event Range
Any adverse event	8 (356,515)	2.77–3.55
Any serious adverse event	5 (356,515)	1.17–1.35
Any adverse event or death	2 (268,701)	1.5–3.37
Arteriovenous fistula	6 (268,701)	<0.1
Cardiac arrest	9 (356,515)	0.26–0.34
Cardiac perforation	7 (268,701)	0.06–0.1
Cardiac valve injury	4 (268,701)	<0.1
Conduction block	6 (268,701)	0.03–0.1
Coronary venous dissection	6 (356,515)	0.08–0.15
Drug reaction	6 (268,701)	0.09–0.11
Hematoma	8 (356,515)	0.84–1.1
Hemothorax	8 (268,701)	0.07–0.1
Infection related to device	6 (268,701)	<0.1
Lead dislodgement	8 (356,515)	0.73–1.2
Myocardial infarction	6 (268,701)	<0.1
Pericardial tamponade	6 (268,701)	0.07–0.1
Peripheral embolism	6 (268,701)	<0.1
Peripheral nerve injury	4 (268,701)	<0.1
Phlebitis, deep	5 (268,701)	<0.1
Phlebitis, superficial	6 (268,701)	0.04–0.1
Pneumothorax	9 (356,515)	0.42–0.51
Stroke/cerebrovascular accident	6 (268,701)	0.05–0.1
Transient ischemic attack	6 (268,701)	<0.1

* Data from Wei, 2011 PMID 21487093 are outliers and are not included. All patients in this study had B-type natriuretic peptide (BNP) measurement which may represent patients with heart failure. Also the study did not explicitly exclude patients with prior ICD.

Table 15. Percentage of patients with late (out of hospital) adverse events and inappropriate shocks (excluding studies of recalled leads or devices)

Outcomes	No. Studies/Cohorts* (N)	Adverse Event Range
Device- and lead-specific adverse events		
Total device-related adverse event	2 (1,820)	4.5-5.2/100 device-mo
ICD mechanical complications	1 (38,992)	4.2%
ICD replacement	3 (5,593)	<0.1-2.6%; 0.1/100 pt-yr
ICD revision	2 (42,245)	2.2-6.4%; 5.2/100 pt-yr
ICD mechanical complication	1 (38,992)	4.2%
Lead-related adverse event, total	3 (15,636)	3.6-5.6%
Lead malfunction	3 (20,242)	2.4-3.9%; 1.14-1.2/100 pt-yr
Lead (high voltage) defect	1 (903)	7.0%
Lead problem requiring surgery	1 (742)	1.8%
Lead failure	3 (4,246)	0.2-3.8%; 1.4/100 pt-yr
Lead fracture requiring revision	1 (1,060)	3.4%
Lead fracture requiring ICD explants	1 (1,339)	<0.1%; 0.07/100 pt-yr
Lead dislodgement	5 (27,084)	0.6-3.1%; 1.4-2.8/100 pt-yr
Lead replacement	3 (15,697)	0.4-1.0%; 0.34-3.4/100 pt-yr
Lead revision or repositioning	5 (12,995)	0.3-19%; 0.8/100 pt-yr
Infection		
Infection, general	2 (199,207)	1.2-2.7%
Infection of ICD device	2 (10,561)	0.9%; 4.2/100 pt-yr
Infection requiring ICD removal	4 (531,959)	0.5-3.7%; 0.7/100 pt-yr
Infection of lead requiring antibiotics	1 (1,060)	0.5%
Infection requiring surgery, nonfatal	1 (742)	0.7%
Pocket infection	1 (667)	1.0%; 1.2/100 pt-yr
Pocket infection requiring debridement	1 (3,340)	1.0%
Sepsis/severe infection	2 (12,868)	0.2% 1st yr: 98.8/100 pt-yr Following: 63.9/100 pt-yr
Thrombosis		
Deep vein thrombosis	1 (38,992)	1.0%
Subclavian vein thrombosis	2 (4,243)	0.2-0.9%
Thromboembolic event, any	1 (681)	2.9%
Inappropriate shocks		
Inappropriate shocks	21 (212,312)	3-21%

ICD = implanted cardiac defibrillator, mo = months; N = number of patients, pt-yr = patient-years.

* Single cohort studies and cohorts (study arms) from comparative studies are counted individually

Table 16. ICDs for Primary Prevention of SCD: Strength of evidence domains

Outcome	Study Design: No. Studies (N)	Study Limitations	Directness	Consistency	Precision	Reporting Bias	Other Issues	Strength of Evidence and Findings
Major outcomes								
Early (in-hospital) AE		Low	Direct	Consistent	Precise	Low	None	High
• Any AE	Registry: 9 (356,515*)							Any AE: 2.8-3.6%
• Serious AE	Registry: 7 (356,515*)							Serious AE: 1.2-1.35%
• Lead dislodgement	RCT:1, Registry: 9 (358,313*)							Lead dislodgement: 0.7-1.2%
• Hematoma	RCT:2, Registry: 9 (360,133*)							Hematoma: 0.8-1.1%
• Multiple†								All other AE: <0.5%
Late (out of hospital) AE		Low	Direct	Inconsistent	Imprecise	Suspected	None	Low
• Total AE‡	RCT: 1 (80)							Total AE§: ICD vs. CRT-D 42% vs. 52% (NS) for 1 yr F/U
• Device-related AE	Cohort: 9 (64,174)							Device-related AE: <0.1-6.4% for 2-49 mo F/U
• Lead-related AE	RCT: 1, Cohort: 23 (57,234*)							Lead-related AE: <0.1-3.9% for 1.5-41 mo F/U
• Infection	Cohort: 15 (65,449*)							Infection: 0.2-3.7% for 1.5-49 mo F/U
• Thrombosis	Cohort: 5 (45,789)							Thrombosis: 0.2-2.9% for 1.5-49 mo F/U
Inappropriate shock	RCT: 1, Cohort: 21 (212,312*)	Low	Direct	Consistent	Imprecise	Low	None	Moderate Inappropriate shock: 3-21% for 1-5y F/U

56

Abbreviations: AE=adverse event; DVT=Deep vein thrombosis; F/U=followup; ICD: implantable cardioverter-defibrillator; mo=month; No.=Number; RCT=randomized, controlled trial; SCD=sudden cardiac death; y=year.

*Largest independent N

† Study design is registry unless otherwise noted. Outcome: No. of studies (largest independent N): Any AE or death: 2 (268,701), Arteriovenous fistula: 7 (268,701), Cardiac arrest: 10 (356,515), Cardiac perforation: 1 RCT, 8 Registry (268,950), Cardiac valve injury: 4(268,701), Conduction block: 7 (268,701), Coronary venous dissection: 2 RCT, 7 Registry (360,133), Drug reaction: 7 (268,701), Hematoma: 1 RCT, 9 Registry (358,335), Hemothorax: 9 (268,701),Hemothorax or pneumothorax: 1 RCT (1798), Infection related to device: 2 RCT, 8 registry (272,319), Myocardial infarction: 7 (268,701), Pericardial tamponade: 7 (268,701), Peripheral embolism: 7 (268,701), Peripheral nerve injury: 5(268,701), Phlebitis – deep: 6(268,701), Phlebitis – superficial: 7 (268,701), Pneumothorax: 2 RCT, 10 Registry (358,584), Pocket problems requiring revision: 1 RCT (1798), Stroke/CVA: 7 (268,701), Transient ischemic attack: 7 (268,701).

‡ Outcome of interest for comparative studies.

§ Left ventricular lead dislodgement, postimplantation left ventricular lead repositioning, permanent failure to deliver biventricular pacing, ventricular tachyarrythmia, hospitalization due to cardiac causes and all-cause mortality.

Figure 10. McHarms quality measures for 38 independent studies reporting adverse event data

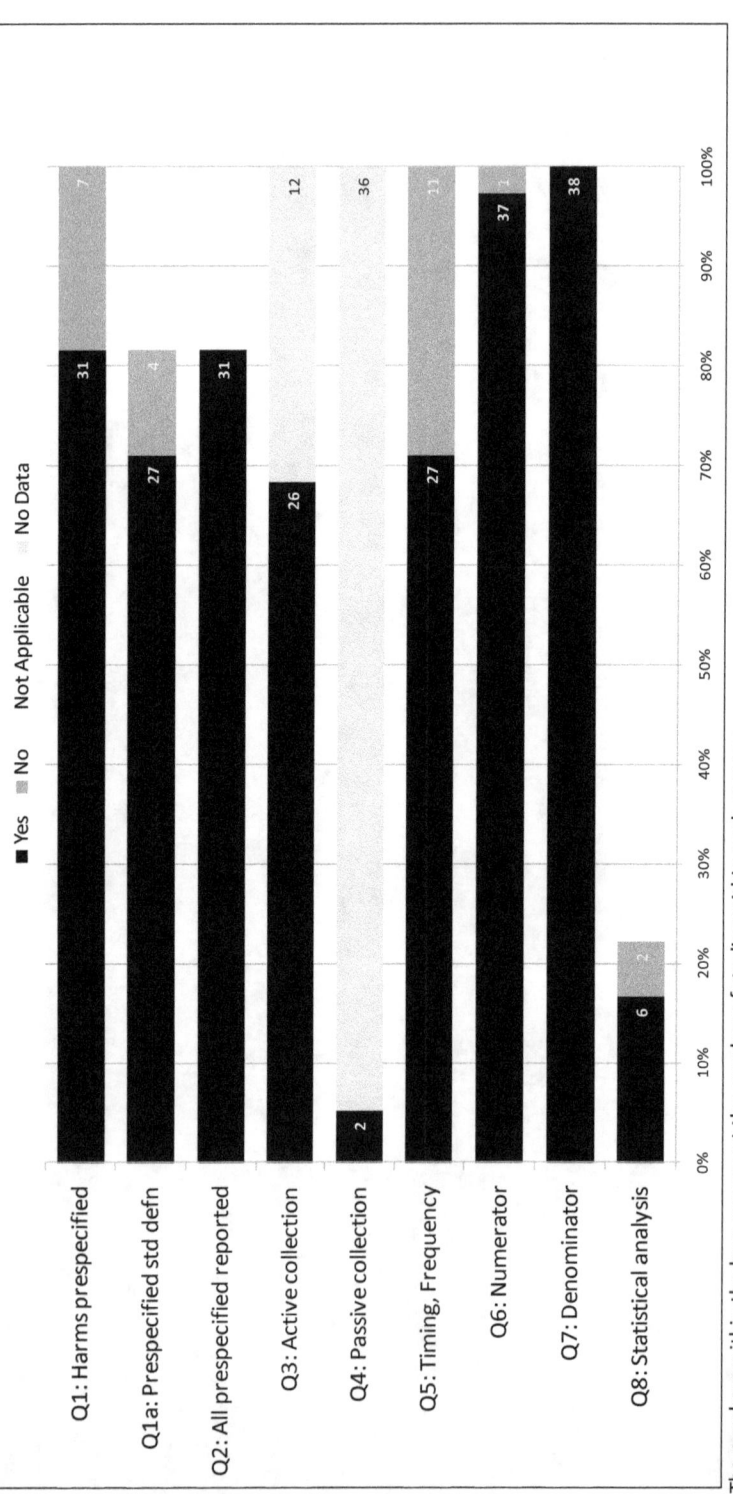

The numbers within the bars represent the number of studies within each category.

Q1. Were any harms prespecified (*a priori*) in Methods section?
Q1a. If yes, were any of them prespecified with *a priori* standardized or precise definitions?
Q2. Were all prespecified harms reported?
Q3. Was the mode of harms collection ACTIVE (sought to collect information on AEs)?
Q4. Was the mode of harms collection PASSIVE? (Participants are not specifically asked about or tested for the occurrence of adverse events. Rather, adverse events are identified based on patient reports made on their own initiative.)
Q5. Did the study specify the TIMING and/or FREQUENCY of collection of harms?
Q6. Is the number of participants who experience harms provided for each arm?
Q7. Is the number at risk for harms (denominator) provided for each arm?
Q8. For studies comparing adverse events across two or more arms: Is there a STATISTICAL analysis of relative harms between groups?

Key Question 3: Which Patients Have Been Included in Comparative Studies of ICDs for Primary Prevention of SCD?

For Key Question 3, we reviewed the eligibility criteria for all 18 studies contributing data to Key Question 1.

Key Question 3a: What Were Eligibility Criteria for Patients in Studies Included for Key Question 1? How Were Patients Evaluated and What Diagnostic Tests and Algorithms Were Used to Select Patients?

Eligibility Criteria

We categorized the studies according to whether they included only a) patients with ischemic cardiomyopathy and MIs that occurred at least 30 days before ICD implantation (henceforth called "remote MIs"), b) patients with nonischemic cardiomyopathy only, c) patients with either ischemic or nonischemic cardiomyopathy and remote MIs, and d) patients with ischemic cardiomyopathy and either MIs that occurred more recently than 30 days before ICD implantation (henceforth called "recent MIs") or coronary revascularization (i.e., patients who would not meet current CMS criteria for ICD implantation for primary prevention of SCD). Note that a study was considered to address remote MI only if all patients had their MI at least 30 days before ICD placement; if the range of timing of MI included some time points of less than 30 days before implantation, the population was considered to have recent MI. **Table 17** provides an overview of the eligibility criteria across studies.

Studies of Patients with Ischemic Cardiomyopathy and Remote MI (>30 days before ICD)

MADIT and MADIT II compared ICD versus no ICD in patients with ischemic cardiomyopathy and remote MI (**Appendix Table 23**).[42,76] Both studies were conducted in the US and Europe. MADIT included adults aged 25 to 80 years; MADIT II included adults over 21 years. Both enrolled only patients in NYHA Classes I, II, and III. The LVEF inclusion criterion for the original MADIT was ≤35 percent. MADIT II was more restrictive, including only those with an LVEF ≤30 percent.

Studies of Patients with Nonischemic Cardiomyopathy

Four studies enrolled patients with nonischemic cardiomyopathy (**Appendix Table 23**).[91,99,103,106] Two RCTs (DEFNITE and CAT) and one nRCS (Fonarow 2000)compared ICD versus no ICD (**Appendix Table 23**).[91,99,106] The third RCT (AMIOVIRT) compared ICD versus amiodarone.[103] The studies of ICD versus no ICD were conducted in the US, and the single study of ICD versus amiodarone was conducted in Germany.

Two studies (CAT and AMIOVIRT) enrolled adults over 18 years of age, but in the CAT study, the upper limit for age was 70 years. The other studies did not set an age restriction for enrollment.

Two RCTs (DEFINITE and AMIOVIRT) enrolled patients in NYHA Classes I, II, and III. The single nRCS (Fonarow 2000) included only those with Classes III and IV. The CAT study restricted its inclusion to those with Classes II and III only.

Two studies (DEFINITE, AMIOVIRT) enrolled only patients with an LVEF ≤35 percent; Fonarow 2000 included patients with LVEF <35 percent. The CAT study was restricted to those with an LVEF ≤30 percent.

Studies of Patients with Mixed Ischemic and Nonischemic Cardiomyopathy

Five RCTs (COMPANION, SCD-HeFT, MADIT-CRT, RAFT and Diab 2011) and three nRCSs (Chan 2009, OPTIMIZE-HF/GWTG-HF, and Mezu 2011) enrolled a mixed population of ischemic and nonischemic cardiomyopathy (**Appendix Table 23**).[51,73,95,105,107,108,112,149] The three nRCSs (Chan 2009, OPTIMIZE-HF/GWTG-HF and Mezu 2011) examined the comparison of ICD versus no ICD,[105,107,108] while a single RCT (SCD-HeFT) compared ICD vs. amiodarone.[7] Another RCT (COMPANION) compared CRT-D versus a control[95] and three additional RCTs (MADIT-CRT, RAFT, and Diab 2011) looked at the comparison of ICD versus CRT-D.[73,112,149] The studies of ICD or CRT-D versus no ICD or amiodarone were conducted in the US. Of the three studies examining ICD versus CRT-D, one was conducted in the US, Canada, and Europe, another in Europe, Canada and Australia, and the third was conducted in the United Kingdom.

One (Chan 2009) of the three nRCSs comparing ICD versus no ICD enrolled patients over 18 years of age. OPTIMIZE-HF/GWTG-HF included patients aged 65 to 84 years while Mezu 2011 restricted its enrollment to only those over 80 years of age. Only one of the RCTs (MADIT-CRT) examining ICD versus CRT-D reported an inclusion criterion for age (> 21 years). COMPANION, RAFT, and SCD-HeFT also did not set an age restriction.

Of the four studies reporting on ICD or CRT-D versus no ICD, two (Chan 2009 and OPTIMIZE-HF/GWTG-HF) did not have an inclusion criterion regarding NYHA class. The remaining two (COMPANION, Mezu 2011) included those with only NYHA Classes III and IV, or Classes I, II, and III respectively. SCD-HeFT included only Classes II and III. One study (MADIT-CRT) of ICD versus CRT-D enrolled only patients in NYHA Classes I and II, while the another enrolled those in NYHA Classes II and III (RAFT), and a third (Diab 2011) enrolled only those in Classes III and IV. In all but two studies, the cutoff for the LVEF was ≤35 percent. The remaining studies (MADIT-CRT and RAFT) were restricted to only patients with an LVEF ≤30 percent. Two RCTs of ICD versus no ICD (COMPANION and Chan 2009) required the patients to have a QRS interval >120 ms. All studies of ICD versus CRT-D set a limit on the QRS interval for enrollment; two (in RAFT and Diab 2011) were ≥120 ms while the other (in MADIT-CRT) was ≥130 ms.

Studies of Patients with Ischemic Cardiomyopathy and Recent MI (<30 days before ICD) or Revascularization

Three RCTs (DINAMIT, IRIS, and MENDMI) enrolled patients with ischemic cardiomyopathy and recent MI (<30 days before ICD implantation)[98,102,111] and a fourth trial (CABG-Patch) enrolled patients with ischemic cardiomyopathy who were undergoing coronary revascularization.[94] The four studies were conducted in multiple countries, including the US and Germany (**Appendix Table 23**). Three (DINAMIT, IRIS, CABG-Patch) had an age restriction as part of their inclusion criteria, enrolling only those younger than 80 years of age.

The three trials of patients with recent MIs (i.e., with at least one patient, but not necessarily all, who had an MI less than 30 days before ICD placement) included those whose MIs occurred either between 6 and 40 days before ICD implantation, 5 and 31 days before, and 3 and 14 days before.

Two studies (DINAMIT and MENDMI) restricted their enrollment by NYHA Class I, II, and III. Three studies (DINAMIT, MENDMI, and CABG-Patch) required an LVEF ≤35 percent, another study (IRIS) included patients with an LVEF ≤40 percent. Two studies specified an inclusion criterion for QRS interval: one (CABG-Patch) set its cutoff at ≥114 ms; the other (MENDMI), <120 ms.

Summary: Eligibility

The two studies of patients with ischemic cardiomyopathy whose MIs occurred at least 30 days prior to ICD implantation included adults with NYHA Class I, II, or III with an LVEF either ≤30 percent or ≤35 percent.

The four studies of patients with nonischemic cardiomyopathy included adults (though one study was restricted to adults 70 years or younger) with a variety of NYHA class criteria. Two RCTs included patients with NYHA Classes I, II, and II; one RCT included only those with Classes II and III; and the nRCS restricted enrollment to Classes III and IV. Three of the studies included patients with LVEF either less than or less than or equal to 35 percent. One trial restricted to LVEF ≤30 percent.

The plurality of studies (five RCTs and two nRCSs) included both patients with ischemic and nonischemic cardiomyopathy. The RCTs included essentially all eligible adults. The two nRCSs, on the other hand, were restricted to older adults, either aged 65 to 84 years or over 80 years. The studies were heterogeneous as to which NYHA Classes were included (I-IV, I-III, I and II, II and III, or III and IV). All but two studies included patients with LVEF either less than or less than or equal to 35 percent; two trial restricted to LVEF ≤30 percent. Four of the trials used QRS interval eligibility criteria of either greater than or greater than or equal to 120 ms or, for one trial, ≥130 ms.

Four trials had eligibility that clearly would not meet current CMS criteria for ICD use for primary prevention of SCD. Three trials included patients with recent MIs, either ≤40, ≤31, or ≤14 days since their MI. The fourth trial was restricted to patients undergoing CABG.

Diagnostic Tests and Algorithms Used to Select Patients

Table 18 displays the diagnostic tests that were used in the RCTs to select patients. No trial explicitly used an algorithm (other than electrophysiology testing, which is described below). All trials used LVEF criteria for eligibility and measured LVEF with a variety of tests, though usually echocardiography; other tests included angiography and radionuclide scanning. All studies except CABG-Patch determined the patients' NYHA class of heart failure. The CRT-D studies and CABG-Patch used QRS intervals on 12-lead electrocardiograms (ECGs) or signal-averaged ECGs; other ICD trials did not.

Six of the 10 ICD versus no ICD trials tested patients for nonsustained VT, most frequently with 24-hour ambulatory Holter monitoring, but also with telemetry, 12-lead ECG, or exercise ECG (stress testing). Only MADIT reported using electrophysiology testing. MADIT II specifically addressed whether electrophysiology testing could be avoided when determining whether ICD placement would be of value.

Only four of the 10 ICD versus no ICD trials and one of the three CRT-D versus ICD trials explicitly tested for coronary stenosis, mostly with coronary angiography or exercise testing. A few trials used other unique diagnostic tests, as listed in **Table 17**.

Summary: Tests Used

There was heterogeneity regarding which diagnostic tests were used to determine study eligibility across trials. (**Table 18**) All RCTs used LVEF criteria, but the studies used different specific tests (though most were based on echocardiography). NYHA class was also determined in all patients (except in one older trial). The trials of CRT-D used QRS interval data for eligibility; most other trials did not. Most of the RCTs of ICD versus no ICD tested all patients for nonsustained VT, but with different specific diagnostic tests. Only one RCT reported performing electrophysiology testing in all patients. Only 4 of the 13 RCTs explicitly tested for coronary stenosis, mostly with coronary angiography or exercise testing.

Key Question 3b: Among Patients in Studies Included for Key Question 1, What Was the Likelihood of SCD or Ventricular Tachyarrhythmia, as Measured by Total Shocks for Those with ICDs or Episodes of SCD for Those without ICDs?

Five RCTs[42,51,94,99,103] and one nRCS (Fonarow 2000[106]) provided data for total shocks or appropriate shocks in patients with an ICD. Some studies provided the data as total number of shocks; others, as number of patients receiving any shock or patients receiving only inappropriate shocks. The data are summarized in **Table 19**. In the first year after ICD implantation, between about one-quarter and one-half of patients had a shock. The percentage of patients who had a shock rose consistently with time since ICD implantation. Four of the studies that reported numbers of shocks (SCD-HeFT, Fonarow 2000, MADIT, CABG-Patch) described the percentage of patients receiving shocks over time and found progressively increasing percentages. Two of the trials (MADIT and CABG-Patch) report survival curves showing that about 50 percent of patients have a shock within the first year, after which the rate of patients having their first shock slows but continues to rise to approximately 70 percent at 4 years (CABG-Patch) and approximately 90 percent at 5 years (MADIT). The studies that reported appropriate shocks revealed similar patterns as for total shocks, though, as expected, with lower rates of appropriate shocks than total shocks.

Six RCTs reported on the episodes of SCDs in patients without an ICD.[42,91,98,99,102,103] CAT reported no SCDs at 1 year. At 2 years, DEFINITE reported episodes in 6.1 percent of patients while MADIT reported episodes in 13 percent. At 3 years, DINAMIT and IRIS reported SCDs in 8.5 and 13 percent of their non-ICD patients, respectively. The study with the longest followup (5 years), AMIOVIRT, reported SCD in only 4 percent of patients at the end of followup. There was no clear trend for increasing likelihood of SCD with longer followup time across the six studies, but within the three RCTs that presented survival curves (DINAMIT, IRIS, and DEFINITE), there appeared to be fairly steady rates of SCD for about 3 to 6 years after randomization.

Summary: Risk of SCD

The six studies that provided data for total or appropriate ICD shocks found that patients in these trials were very likely to have a shock during followup. The majority of the first episodes of being shocked appear to occur within the first year after ICD implantation. The six RCTs that reported SCD in patients without an ICD included with a likelihood of SCD between about 4 and 13 percent during the 2 to 5 years after randomization. Rates of SCD over time appeared to be fairly steady.

Table 17. Eligibility criteria in comparative study

Study Author Year	IDCM & Documented MI	NIDCM >3 mo	NYHA II/III	NYHA IV/CRT	LVEF ≤35%	No MI <40 d	No Revasc <3 mo	No shock / hTN	Revasc not indicated	No brain damage	Exp Surv >1 y
ICD vs. No ICD											
AMIOVIRT Strickberger 2003	--	Yes (no time*)	No (also Class I)	--	Yes	Yes (implied)	Yes (implied)	nd	Yes	nd	nd
CABG-Patch Bigger 1997	No (MI not required)	--	nd	nd	Yes	nd	No	nd	No (al having CABG)	nd	Yes
CAT Bänsch 2002	--	No (≤9 mo)	Yes	--	Yes	Yes	Yes (implied)	nd	Yes	nd	nd
Chan 2009	Yes	Yes	nd	nd	Yes	No (No MI <30 d)	Yes (no time*)	nd	nd	nd	Yes
COMPANION Bristow 2004	No (MI not required)	Yes (no time*)	Yes	Yes	Yes	nd	nd	nd	nd	nd	nd
DEFINITE Kadish 2004	--	Yes (no time*)	No (also Class I)	--	Yes	Yes (implied)	Yes (implied)	nd	Yes	nd	nd
DINAMIT Hohnloser 2004	Yes	--	No (also Class I)	--	Yes	No (All MI ≤40 d)	Yes (implied)	nd	Yes	nd	Yes ("limited")
Fonarow 2000	--	Yes (no time*)	Yes	Maybe (nd re: CRT)	Yes	Yes	Yes (implied)	nd	nd	nd	nd
IRIS Steinbeck 2009	Yes	--	No (also Class I)	--	No (≤40%)	No (All MI ≤31 d)	nd	nd	Yes	nd	Yes ("severe")
MADIT Moss 1996	Yes	--	No (also Class I)	--	Yes	No (No MI <21 d)	No (<2 mo)	nd	Yes	Yes	Yes
MADIT II Moss 2002	Yes	--	No (also Class I)	--	Yes	No (No MI <1 mo)	Yes	Yes	Yes	Yes	Yes
Mezu 2011	No (MI not required)	Yes (no time*)	No (also Class I)	--	Yes	No (any time)	No (implied)	nd	No (implied)	No	No
OPTIMIZE-HF / GWTG-HF Hernandez 2010	No (MI not required)	Yes (no time*)	nd	nd	Yes	nd	nd	nd	nd	nd	nd
SCD-HeFT Bardy 2005	No (MI not required)	Yes (no time*)	Yes	--	Yes	nd	nd	nd	nd	nd	nd
ICD vs. CRT-D											
Diab 2011	No (MI not required)	Yes (no time*)	Yes	Yes	Yes	nd	nd	nd	Yes	nd	No (>6 mo)
MADIT-CRT Moss 2009	Yes	Yes	No (also Class I)	--	Yes	Yes	Yes	nd	Yes	Yes	Yes
MENDMI Chung 2010	Yes	--	No (also Class I)	--	Yes	No (all MI ≤14 d)	Yes	nd	nd	nd	No (>6 mo)

64

Study Author Year	IDCM & Documented MI	NIDCM >3 mo	NYHA II/III	NYHA IV/CRT	LVEF ≤35%	No MI <40 d	No Revasc <3 mo	No shock / hTN	Revasc not indicated	No brain damage	Exp Surv >1 y
RAFT Tang, 2010 21073365	No (MI not required)	Yes	Yes	--	Yes	nd	nd	nd	nd	nd	nd

Explanation of headers:

IDCM & Documented MI: Ischemic dilated cardiomyopathy and documented prior myocardial infarction

NIDCM >3 mo: Nonischemic dilated cardiomyopathy >3 months (with or without prior myocardial infarction)

NYHA II/III: New York Heart Association Class II or III heart failure

NYHA IV/CRT: NYHA Class IV heart failure and meet all current CMS coverage requirements for a cardiac resynchronization therapy device

LVEF ≤35%: Left ventricular ejection fraction ≤35%

No MI <40 d: No acute myocardial infarction within the past 40 days

No Revasc <3 mo: No coronary artery revascularization (coronary artery bypass graft or percutaneous transluminal coronary angioplasty) within the past 3 months

No shock / hTN: No cardiogenic shock or symptomatic hypotension while in a stable baseline rhythm

Revasc not indicated: No clinical symptoms or findings that would make them a candidate for coronary revascularization

No brain damage: No irreversible brain damage from preexisting cerebral disease

Exp Surv >1 y: No disease, other than cardiac disease (e.g. cancer, uremia, liver failure), associated with a likelihood of survival <1 year

Abbreviations: -- = this factor was not part of inclusion criteria (e.g., AMIOVIRT trial excluded patients with ischemic dilated cardiac disease), CABG = coronary artery bypass graft, CRT-D = cardiac resynchronization therapy and implanted cardioverter defibrillator, ICD = implanted cardioverter defibrillator, nd = not documented.

* Eligibility criteria did not include duration of NIDCM or time since revascularization

65

Table 18. Diagnostic tests used to select patients (RCTs only)*

Study	LVEF Measured (Test)	QRS Measured	NYHA Class Determined	NSVT	EP Study	Coronary Stenosis (Test)	Other
ICD vs. No ICD							
AMIOVIRT / Strickberger 2003	Yes (nd)	No	Yes	Yes (multiple†)	No	Yes, implied (nd)	No
CABG-Patch / Bigger 1997	Yes (nd)	Yes (SA ECG)	No	No	No	Yes, implied (angiography)	No
CAT / Bänsch 2002	Yes (angiography)	No	Yes	Yes (Holter)	No	Yes (angiography)	No
COMPANION / Bristow 2004	Yes (echo)	Yes (ECG)	Yes	No	No	No	No
DEFINITE / Kadish 2004	Yes (nd)	No	Yes	Yes (Holter or telemetry)	No	Yes (angiography or ETT)	No
DINAMIT / Hohnloser 2004	Yes (multiple‡)	No	Yes	No	No	No	RR interval (Holter)
IRIS / Steinbeck 2009	Yes (echo)	No	Yes	Yes (Holter)	No	No	No
MADIT / Moss 1996	Yes (multiple‡)	No	Yes	Yes (multiple§)	Yes	No	No
MADIT II / Moss 2002	Yes (multiple‡)	No	Yes	No	No	No	No
SCD-HeFT / Bardy 2005	Yes (nd)	No	Yes	Yes (Holter)	No	No	6 min walk, CXR
ICD vs. CRT-D							
Diab 2011	Yes (echo)	Yes (nd)	Yes	No	No	Yes (ETT)	Mech dyssynch (echo or TDI) LVEDD (echo)
MADIT-CRT / Moss 2009	Yes (echo)	Yes (nd)	Yes	No	No	No	No
MENDMI / Chung 2010	Yes (echo)	Yes (ECG)	Yes	No	No	No	WMA (echo) 6-min walk
RAFT / Tang, 2010 21073365	Yes (nd)	Yes (nd)	Yes	No	No	No	No

6 min walk = 6 minute walk test, CRT-D = cardiac resynchronization therapy with defibrillator, CXR = chest radiography, ECG = electrocardiography, Echo = echocardiography, EP = electrophysiology, ETT = exercise tolerance test (stress test), Holter = 24-hour Holter monitor, ICD = implanted cardiac defibrillator, LVEDD = left ventricle end-diastolic diameter, LVEF = left ventricle ejection fraction, nd = not documented, Mech dyssynch = mechanical ventricular dyssynchrony, NSVT = nonsustained ventricular tachycardia, NYHA = New York Heart Association, SA ECG = signal averaged ECG, RR interval = time between R waves on ECG, TDI = tissue Doppler imaging, WMA = left ventricular wall motion abnormality.

* Excluding laboratory tests, symptoms, past medical history, or physical examination findings.
† ECG, telemetry or Holter monitor
‡ Angiography, radionuclide scanning, or echocardiography
§ ECG, Holter, or exercise ECG.

Table 19. Patients with any shock from ICD and sudden cardiac deaths (with no ICD)

Study Author, Year PMID, Country	Intervention (Control)	Patients with an ICD who received any shock [appropriate shocks]	Patients with no ICD with SCD
5 y			
AMIOVIRT Strickberger, 2003 12767651, US	ICD (Amiodarone)	nd total [31% [16/51] appropriate]	3.8% (2/52)
4 y			
SCD-HeFT Bardy, 2005 15659722, US	ICD (Amiodarone)	31% (259/829) any shock; 7.5%/y [21% (177/829) appropriate; 5.1%/y]	nd
3 y			
DINAMIT Hohnloser, 2004 15590950, Multi	ICD (No ICD)	nd	8.5%; 3.5%/y (29/342)
IRIS Steinbeck, 2009 19812399, Germany	ICD (No ICD)	nd	13.2% (60/453)
2 y			
CABG-Patch Bigger, 1997 9371853, US and Germany	ICD (No ICD)	57% actuarial risk (N=428) any shock	nd
DEFINITE Kadish, 2004 15152060, US	ICD (No ICD)	nd any shock* [18% (41/229) appropriate]	6.1% (14/229)
Fonarow, 2000 10760339, US	ICD (Control)	nd any shock† [40% (10/25) appropriate (55% actuarial risk)]	nd
MADIT Moss, 1996 8960472, US and EU	ICD (No ICD)	60% (54/90) any shock	12.9% (13/101)
1 y			
CAT Bänsch, 2002 11914254, Germany	ICD (Control)	nd	0% (0/50)
CABG-Patch Bigger, 1997 9371853, US and Germany	ICD (No ICD)	50% actuarial risk (N=428) any shock	nd
Fonarow, 2000 10760339, US	ICD (Control)	27% actuarial risk (N=25) any shock	nd

1°=primary, CABG=coronary artery bypass graft, EU=Europe, ICD=implantable cardiac defibrillator, LVEF=left ventricular ejection fraction, MI=myocardial infarction, nd=not documented, NYHA=New York Heart Association, RCT=randomized controlled trial, UK, United Kingdom, US=United States.

* 49 patients received inappropriate shocks; no data on how many patients in any shock received shocks.
† 3 patients received inappropriate shocks; no data on how many patients in any shock received shocks.

Discussion

Key Findings and Strength of Evidence

We identified 14 studies comparing ICD versus no ICD, 4 studies comparing CRT-D versus ICD, and 59 studies contributing data on adverse events after ICD implantation. The summary of key findings and strength of evidence is shown in **Table 20**. This table is an amalgamation of Tables 3, 7, and 10, plus outcomes with insufficient evidence.

Table 20. Summary of findings

Outcome	Study Design: No. Studies (N)	Findings	Strength of Evidence
All-cause mortality	ICD vs. no ICD RCT: 10 (8,606) nRCS: 4 (5,949)	• ICD use as primary prevention for patients who meet the current practice criteria (no recent MI, no concurrent coronary revascularization) reduces the risk of all-cause mortality over the course of 3 to 7 years after implantation: HR = 0.69 (95% CI 0.60, 0.79). The benefit of ICD appears fairly stable over time. Across trials, the range of NNT to prevent one death was 6.2 to 22 at 3 to 7 years, with wide 95% CIs. • There is indirect evidence across studies that patients with recent MIs (<30-40 days), on average, do not benefit from ICD, in contrast with patients with more distant MIs. • Within-study subgroup analyses fail to support whether the value of ICD placement differs in other subgroups of patients, including by sex or age, or based on different characteristics of facilities where ICDs are implanted.	High
	CRT-D vs. ICD RCT: 4 (3,743)	• The 2 larger trials found either no difference (HR = 1.00) or a significant benefit with CRT-D (HR = 0.75)No differences in effect were found between patients with ischemic or nonischemic heart disease or with NYHA Class II or III cardiomyopathy • There was no evidence regarding the comparison of CRT-D and ICD in subgroups of patients or based on different characteristics of facilities where ICDs are implanted.	Insufficient
Sudden cardiac death	ICD vs. no ICD RCT: 7 (4,093)nRCS: 2 (1,115)	• ICD use as primary prevention for patients who meet the current practice criteria (no recent MI, no concurrent coronary revascularization) reduces the risk of SCD over the course of 2 to 6 years after implantation: HR = 0.37 (95% CI 0.26, 0.52). There is insufficient evidence to evaluate the course of the effect over time. Across trials, the range of NNT to prevent one SCD was approximately 2.0 to 11. • Within-study subgroup analyses fail to support whether the value of ICD placement differs in subgroups of patients or based on different characteristics of facilities where ICDs are implanted.	High

Outcome	Study Design: No. Studies (N)	Findings	Strength of Evidence
Sustained ventricular tachyarrhythmia	0	• There is no evidence	Insufficient
Quality of life	ICD vs. no ICD RCT: 3 (1,825)	• The evidence failed to show a consistent effect of ICD placement on quality of life. • There is no evidence regarding subgroups.	Low
Early AEs (In-hospital)	RCT: 3 (3,867) Observational: 11 (356,515[†]) [overlapping cohorts]	• During hospitalization, 2.8–3.6% of patients have any adverse event. Serious adverse events occurred in 1.2–1.35% after ICD placement. • The most common specific adverse events were lead dislodgement (0.7–1.2%) and hematoma (0.8–1.1%). Other in-hospital adverse events occurred in ≤0.5% of patients receiving ICDs • Based on within-study subgroups analyses, there may be higher rates of adverse events among patients receiving dual-chamber ICDs, CRT-D, among older patients, women, and those with ESRD. Physicians and hospitals with lower volume of implantation and operators other than electrophysiologists may have more adverse events.	High
Late AEs (Out of hospital)	RCT: 3 (2,149) Observational: 28 reports of 22 independent cohorts (99,725[‡])	• Device-related adverse events occurred in <0.1–6.4% of ICD patients during 2–49 month followup. • Other relatively common adverse events included lead malfunction (<0.1–3.9% during 1.5–40 month followup), infection (0.2–3.7% for 1.5–49 month followup), and thrombosis (0.2–2.9% for 1.5–49 month followup). • Based on within-study subgroup analyses, there may be more lead-related adverse events in women. There was no apparent difference in adverse events between CRT-D and ICD or between dual and single chamber ICDs.	Low
Inappropriate shock	RCT: 1 (249) Observational: 21 reports of 17 independent cohorts (212,063§)	• Inappropriate shock occurred in 3–21% of patients during 1–5 year followup. • Based on within-study subgroup analyses, there may be more inappropriate shocks among younger patients. There were mixed data on the difference in inappropriate shocks between dual and single chamber ICDs. Limited data show no apparent difference in inappropriate shocks between CRT-D and ICD, or between dual and single chamber ICDs.	Moderate

AE = adverse event, CI = confidence interval, CMS = Centers for Medicare and Medicaid Services, CRT-D = cardiac resynchronization therapy-defibrillator, ESRD = end stage renal disease, HR = hazard ration, ICD = implantable cardioverter–defibrillator, MI = myocardial infarction, No. =number, nRCS = nonrandomized comparative study, NYHA = New York Heart Association, RCT = randomized, controlled trial, SCD = sudden cardiac death.

† Largest independent N

‡ Largest independent N. Two large cohorts: N=38,992 (PMID 21795298), N=15,387 (PMID 19925609).

§ Largest independent N. One large cohort N=185,778 (PMID 21098452)

Overall, there is a high strength of evidence, with the RCTs and nRCSs showing a consistent and precise benefit of all-cause mortality reduction in selected patients undergoing ICD implantation for primary prevention of SCD compared to those being treated without ICD. The patients who benefit have a combination of reduced LVEF, nonischemic cardiomyopathy and heart failure or a combination of reduced LVED, ischemic cardiomyopathy and at least 30 to 40 days after a MI or 3 months after revascularization. Meta-analysis of seven RCTs yielded a HR of 0.69 (95% CI 0.60, 0.79) for death. Followup ranged from 3 to 7 years. The reported Kaplan Meier curves generally found that the reduction in all-cause mortality with ICD was fairly stable over time. Across RCTs, the NNT to prevent one death at ranged from 6.2 (95% CI 4.0, 18) to 22 (95% CI 2.3, infinite) at the longest durations of followup (3 to 7 years). Three studies of patients who were not in the selected populations because their ICDs were implanted immediately after MI (IRIS[102] and DINAMIT[98]) or were undergoing CABG (CABG-Patch[163]) did not show a benefit with respect to all-cause mortality. Regarding the outcome SCD, meta-analysis of five studies (again excluding IRIS and DINAMIT) showed benefit from ICD use for reducing SCD (HR 0.37; 95% CI 0.26, 0.52) over the course of 2 to 6 years after implantation. Across RCTs, the NNT to prevent one arrhythmic death ranged from about 2 to 3 (approximate 95% CI 1.3, 16) to 11 (95% CI 1.3, infinite). The evidence suggests that the effect of ICD versus no ICD on SCD over time may increase beyond 2 or 3 years. The finding of a large benefit on SCD, which increased over time, contrasts with a smaller benefit for all-cause mortality, which remained constant over time. This suggests that there are competing risks for mortality in this population limiting the effectiveness of ICDs to reduce death.

Three RCTs of ICD versus no ICD examined QoL with a broad range of QoL measures, but no specific QoL measure was evaluated by more than a single trial. Two of the trials found no difference in QoL with various QoL tools (Health Utility Index 3, Quality of Well-being Schedule, and the State Trait Anxiety Inventory). The third trial found differences favoring no ICD for 2 out of 7 specific components of SF-36 and for perception of health transition. However, this latter trial is of limited applicability to current practice, both because all patients had CABG and because the trial implanted epicardial ICD systems which are much more invasive compared to the transvenous ICDs currently employed. Thus, given the sparseness of data on QoL and the lack of consistency across trials, overall, there is a low strength of evidence low strength of evidence that failed to show a consistent effect of ICD placement on QoL. There is insufficient evidence to evaluate differential effects of ICD on QoL in different populations of patients or based on different characteristics of facilities where ICDs are implanted.

Our analyses failed to show statistically significant differences for all-cause mortality or SCD across subgroups, including by meta-analysis. This contrasts with conclusions by others who proposed differential effects by age and sex. Two prior reviews have proposed no or less benefit from ICDs in women.[164,165] One other review concluded that ICDs may be less effective in older adults.[172] We believe that these conclusions were based on an over-reliance of within subgroup findings despite nonsignificant interaction tests, study selection (the MUSTT trial included in the review by Ghanbari was unfavorable for women), and lower precision due to women constituting only 23 percent of the study populations.[164,166] Our Table 5 and Figures 6 and 7 indicate that the studies consistently found no significant difference in effect between men and women (or other subgroups of patients). However there may be an indication that ICDs are more effective in patients with more distant coronary revascularization compared with recent surgery. Indirect review across studies suggests that patients with recent MIs (within 31 or 40 days) have no reduction in all-cause mortality in contrast with patients with more distant MIs. The evidence fails to support a difference in the benefit of ICD based on time since MI, coronary revascularization, or kidney disease. There is insufficient evidence to evaluate differential effects of ICD on all-cause mortality or SCD in based on different characteristics of clinicians implanting ICDs or facilities where ICDs are implanted. Four RCTs examined the effect of adding CRT to ICD versus ICD alone. Two trials were too small to yield meaningful conclusions regarding death.[111,112] MADIT-CRT[167] found no difference in all-cause death in patients with ischemic or nonischemic cardiomyopathy. In contrast, RAFT found a significant 25 percent reduction in all-cause death with CRT-D in patients with NYHA Class II or III cardiomyopathy (but no difference in effect between Class II and III).[149] Given the inconsistencies between the two studies, there is insufficient evidence regarding how CRT-D and ICD alone compare to prevent all-cause death. Our review examined whether the addition of CRT to ICD impacts mortality. It is important to note that we did not include the review of other outcomes that may be affected by CRT, such as heart failure and related hospitalizations.

We found no study specifically examining the effect of ICD with ATP versus ICD alone for primary prevention. A prior trial compared ICDs with and without ATP for primary or secondary prevention patients and showed benefit for QOL.[57] ATP is now a standard software feature available in all modern transvenous ICD systems and can be readily activated by a clinician if deemed appropriate for any given patient. Thus the question of ATP versus no ATP is not as relevant. Instead the more important programming features which have been elucidated by MADIT-RIT are those of rate cut-off and detection delay in addition to the use of ATP.[168] MADIT-RIT is discussed in detail below in the section on excluded studies.

We reviewed study eligibility criteria and how the criteria compare to current CMS coverage criteria. Several trials excluded older adults (>70 years to 84 years), whereas two nRCSs included only older adults 65 to 84 years or ≥80 years. All studies used a LVEF criterion but different methods of ascertainment of the EF. IRIS[102] included patients with a LVEF <40 percent, but all other studies included only those with LVEF≤35 percent . The actual mean LVEF at baseline in all studies was below 30 percent. The studies were heterogeneous as to which NYHA Classes (I-IV) were included. The three trials comparing CRT-D versus ICD used QRS interval criteria which varied from≥130 ms in MADIT -CRT[167] ≥120 ms in Diab[112] 2011 and <120 ms in MENDMI.[111] Other approaches to risk stratification for SCD prior to ICD implantation varied across studies. MADIT was the only study that used formal electrophysiological testing.

Although this report's Key Questions did not cover the comparison of the patients in the eligible trials and patients enrolled in the National Cardiovascular Data Registry ICD Registry (NCDR), a recent publication partially does so for patients undergoing primary prevention ICD placement.[169] Masoudi et al. provide baseline characteristics data for NCDR, MADIT II, and SCD-HeFT. Although, they did not conduct direct comparisons, notable differences between the trials and NCDR include less frequent NYHA Class III (MADIT II 25% and SCD-HeFT 30%; NCDR 52%), less frequent hypertension (MADIT II 53% and SCD-HeFT 55%; NCDR 75%), less common LBBB (MADIT II 19%; NCDR 29%), and more digoxin use (MADIT II 57% and SCD-HeFT 67%; NCDR 29%). Compared to NCDR, the patients in the trials also had lower mean age (MADIT II 64 years and SCD-HeFT 60 years; NCDR 68 years), lower percentage of women (MADIT II 16% and SCD-HeFT 23%; NCDR 27%), and LVEF (MADIT II 23% and SCD-HeFT 24%; NCDR 25%),.

Six RCTs reported SCD in the control groups that were not assigned to ICD. They found SCD occurring in 4 to 13 percent of patients during 2 to 5 years after randomization. There was no clear trend for increasing rates of SCD with longer followup.

The benefits of ICDs have to be weighed against the risks. A high strength of evidence shows overall early in-hospital adverse event rates ranging from 2.8 to 3.6 percent and serious adverse event rates ranging from 1.2 to 1.35 percent. The most common early adverse events are lead dislodgement (in 0.73 to 1.2% of patients) and hematoma (in 0.84 to 1.1% of patients). Higher rates of in-hospital adverse events have been shown in the following subgroups: patients implanted with dual-chamber ICDs or CRT-Ds (vs. single-chamber ICDs); patients who are older, female, or have ESRD; patients implanted by physicians with a lower implantation volume or by nonelectrophysiologists; and patients implanted at hospitals with a lower implantation volume.

Regarding late (out of hospital) adverse events, there is low strength of evidence that device-related adverse events (with variable definitions) occurred in <0.1 to 6.4 percent of patients for followup durations of 2 to 49 months. Lead-related adverse events occurred in <0.1 to 3.9 percent of patients with followup durations from 1.5 to 40 months, but in 7.0 to 19 percent of patients during longer followup (35 to 96 months). Based on moderate strength evidence, the percentage of patients who experienced at least one inappropriate shock ranged from 3 to 21 percent for followup between 1 and 5 years.

Generally, these risks from ICD identified in this review appear low. However, it is possible there is underreporting for hospital based complications, and a gross underestimation of complications after hospital discharge which are not systematically captured.

Comparison With Current Knowledge

Our findings for benefit from ICD implantation for primary prevention of SCD are consistent with those in the literature. A prior meta-analysis of the same seven RCTs we combined in our main analysis found a HR of 0.74 (95% CI 0.67, 0.83).[170] This estimate differs slightly from our estimate due to selecting different control arms from COMPANION[95] and SCD-HeFT.[51] Another meta-analysis restricted to five trials in individuals with nonischemic cardiomyopathy found a HR for mortality of 0.69 (95% CI 0.55, 0.87).[171]

The studies in our review failed to find statistically significant differences in effects across subgroups. Two prior reviews concluded that ICDs were ineffective or less effective in women and older adults.[164,165,172] However, these conclusions are based on a faulty reliance on nonstatistically significant findings in *post hoc* subgroups with relatively small sample sizes (women and older adults).

A retrospective cohort study of Medicare beneficiaries hospitalized with heart failure and LVEF ≤35 percent who were selected for ICD therapy had lower risk-adjusted long-term mortality compared with those who did not receive an ICD.[107] This study is susceptible to bias by indication.

Supplementary Evidence in Excluded Studies

Additional studies that did not meet inclusion criteria for our review supplement our findings. MUSTT was not included in the review, as it was not designed with the specific intention to test ICD therapy versus no ICD therapy for the primary prevention of SCD.[41] It compared treatment administered according to a risk stratification algorithm with electrophysiological testing, followed by antiarrhythmic therapy or ICD in those who failed antiarrhythmic therapy versus routine medical management without antiarrhythmic therapy. The risk of cardiac arrest or death from arrhythmia among the patients who received an ICD was significantly lower than that among the patients receiving no antiarrhythmic therapy (adjusted risk ratio [RR] 0.27; 95% CI 0.15, 0.47). The risk of death from all-causes was also significantly lower in patients who received an ICD than in those who received no antiarrhythmic therapy (adjusted RR 0.45; 95%

CI 0.32, 0.63). Those receiving medical antiarrhythmic therapy had the highest risk of all-cause mortality and SCD. The trial provided evidence that electrophysiologically guided antiarrhythmic therapy with ICDs reduces the risk of SCD in high-risk patients with CAD, LVEF ≤40 percent, spontaneous and unsustained VT, or sustained tachyarrhythmia induced by programmed stimulation.

Another study in individuals undergoing ICD implantation for primary prevention, MADIT-RIT, did not meet criteria for inclusion in Key Question 1, as it assessed the effect of different programming algorithms to avoid inappropriate ATP or shock therapy.[60] However, the trial's data on inappropriate shocks were included in the evidence base for Key Question 2. MADIT-RIT compared three arms with different programming approaches: one with higher rate cutoffs (with a 2.5 second delay before the initiation of therapy at a heart rate of ≥200 beats per minute), one of programming with longer delays (with a 60 second delay at 170 to 199 beats per minute, a 12 second delay at 200 to 249 beats per minute, and a 2.5 second delay at ≥250 beats per minute), and one of conventional programming (with a 2.5 second delay at 170 to 199 beats per minute and a 1.0 second delay at ≥200 beats per minute). The primary outcome measure was time to the first occurrence of inappropriate therapy, either inappropriate ATP or shock, and the secondary outcomes were all-cause mortality and syncope. The trial showed that programming a higher rate cutoff or a longer delay prior to ATP or shock therapy resulted in a lower rate of inappropriate therapy compared with conventional programming. Both interventional arms also had lower mortality for high-rate therapy versus conventional therapy (HR 0.45; 95% CI 0.24, 0.85 for high-rate therapy vs. conventional therapy; and HR 0.56; 95% CI 0.30, 1.02 for delayed therapy versus conventional therapy).

With regard to trials of CRT-D versus ICD, we did not include the Multicenter InSync ICD Randomized Clinical Evaluation trial (MIRACLE ICD),[173] the cardiac resynchronization therapy for the treatment of heart failure in patients with intraventricular conduction delay and malignant ventricular tachyarrhythmias trial (CONTAK-CD),[88] since these trials were not exclusively primary prevention trials. Although the Cardiac-Resynchronization Therapy in Heart Failure with Narrow QRS Complexes trial (RETHINQ) evaluated CRT-D versus ICD therapy, it was also not included in our review as there were no outcomes of interest.[174]

Applicability

The review of the eligibility criteria shows that the findings are applicable to selected individuals in the US and other high-resource countries, in particular individuals with nonischemic or ischemic cardiomyopathy and reduced LVEF (<30 to 35%). For patients with ischemic cardiomyopathy, the finding of benefit from ICD applies to those more than 30 to 40 days after MI and at least 3 months after revascularization.

Compared with the population of primary prevention therapy in the NCDR, the RCT populations of key trials were younger, less often women, and had had a lower burden of comorbidity.[169] The subgroup analyses showed no evidence to suggest different efficacy of ICDs in women or older adults. Nevertheless, how representative the trial findings are to the larger eligible Medicare population is an important question. Five out of seven comparative studies in the review provided subgroup data for those over 65 years. They showed that about a third to half of patients were 65 years or older, while the proportion in NCDR is well over 42%.[175] One cohort study followed Medicare Beneficiaries (median age 75 years) after primary ICD implantation and found a mortality at 3 years of follow up of 31%.[176] This was higher than in the major primary ICD trials SCD-HEFT (mean age 60 years, 3 year mortality 16%) and MADIT-II (mean age 64 years, three year mortality 22%). However, almost half of the Medicare patients did not have previous heart failure hospitalizations and received an ICD on the admission day suggesting they were electively admitted for the procedure. In this subgroup, the mortality of 22% was similar to that of the large trials, despite the difference in mean ages. While most trials did not specify that patients were electively admitted for ICD implantation, this is assumed to be the case.[176] This suggests that the trial findings may apply to a sizeable proportion of Medicare patients.

The estimates for adverse events derive from studies with mixed populations (i.e., patients who received ICDs for primary or secondary prevention). One study found no statistically significant difference in the risk of an adverse event or death between patients with ICDs for primary and those with ICDs for secondary prevention, supporting the notion that the rate of procedure-related adverse events, which contribute the majority of adverse events, may be similar across primary and secondary populations.[117]

Limitations

Limitations of the evidence base in some RCTs include lack of blinding of outcome assessors of arrhythmia outcomes or SCD, high attrition rates (>20%), or differential rates of attrition and/or crossover between study groups and differences in the control treatments or in the rates of concomitant use of beta blockers between the study groups. Of note, all trials conducted intention-to-treat analyses. Nonsignificant subgroup analyses need to be interpreted in the context of studies likely being underpowered to explore differences in effects across subgroups of interest. At the same time, positive treatment effects within subgroups may represent spurious findings from multiple testing. The quality of the long-term adverse events suffered from a lack of harmonized definitions and systematic ascertainment. This review does not provide a complete assessment of the effectiveness of CRT. The intention of ICD therapy is restoration of normal sinus rhythm in the setting of life-threatening arrhythmias, and the intention of CRT is improvement of functional status and symptoms of heart failure. We did not include heart failure outcomes, which were primary outcomes of interest for the studies comparing CRT-D versus ICD as the focus of our review was prevention of SCD rather than management of heart failure. It is important to point out that study populations in ICD trials and CRT trials have overlapping characteristics but are not exactly the same. Research Gaps

The gaps in our current knowledge are large with regard to knowing which patients should be offered ICD with the expectation of improving meaningful survival. The rates of SCD in the non-ICD trial arms were not consistently reported. Consistent reporting would facilitate an assessment of how the mortality benefit may be correlated with the baseline risk. There is a great need for better risk stratification tools and their validation to better identify those patients who are most likely to benefit from ICD therapy. Some risk scores have been developed in clinical trials and may be used going forward towards reducing the risk of unnecessary ICD implantation. However, since most sudden deaths are not in patients with previously identified risk factors, there is a need explore risk prediction tools that extend beyond currently used trial inclusion criteria.

While it is beyond the scope of the current report, additional risk stratification tools are continually being examined, including measures of autonomic function such as T-wave alternans. This latter modality has been formally studied in a comparative analysis with EP testing in the ABCD (Alternans Before Cardioverter Defibrillator) Trial.[177] In addition, advances in magnetic resonance imaging (MRI) or genetic testing may be useful in the future.

Similarly, analyses of subgroups of patients who may particularly benefit (or derive no benefit) from ICD use are needed, especially when the etiology, pathophysiology and competing risks for death differ.To date, the analyses of subgroups are underpowered and inconclusive. A patient-level meta-analysis across major trials may be able to provide the power to adequately evaluate subgroups. Future trials should focus on elderly, women, who constitute only a minority in clinical ICD trials, and on patients with chronic kidney disease. We found no eligible studies in children, pointing to this group also requiring future study.

A research gap also exists in the area of primary prevention of SCD in familial or inherited conditions as well as less common cardiomyopathies including but not limited to long-QT syndrome, Brugada syndrome, catecholaminergic polymorphic VT, hypertrophic cardiomyopathy, arrhythmogenic right ventricular dysplasia, cardiac sarcoidosis, and left ventricle noncompaction. These disease states are less prevalent than ischemic cardiomyopathy and nonischemic dilated cardiomyopathy and were, in large part, implicitly or explicitly excluded from the studies in this review. In particular, patients with channelopathies have structurally normal hearts (i.e., those with normal LVEFs) but nonetheless, may have an elevated risk of SCD. Patients with hypertrophic cardiomyopathy generally have hyperdynamic ventricles until they reach the end stage of the disease process. Thus, many or most of these patients would have also been excluded in the RCTs to date. While there are research gaps for these patient groups, the low prevalence of some of these diseases presents challenges for conducting RCTs. The NCDR ICD database provides an opportunity to track these patients and describe their outcomes.

As mentioned above, the intent of this review was to address sudden cardiac death outcomes rather than heart failure outcomes. Since one of the primary goals of chronic resynchronization therapy is the improvement of heart failure, this issue was not completely addressed. Thus, a comparative effectiveness review of CRT warrants a separate review in order to address outcomes related to heart failure and mortality. In order to be comprehensive, CRT-P and CRT-D studies have to be included.

While there is robust information on adverse events immediately post implantation in the hospital, there are also large gaps in the knowledge about adverse events after the hospitalization for implantation and the impact on patient reported outcomes. This includes information on likelihood of lead complications needing revision, likelihood of both appropriate and inappropriate shocks, resulting distress from ICD shocks and impact on QoL. Another crucial issue that is uncertain is the impact of ICD on the quality of death, and the challenge to approach ICD inactivation to avoid undesired shocks at the end of life.

In an era of fast-paced technological advances, it is imperative to critically reevaluate the incremental net benefit and cost of evolving medical and device therapies. On September 28, 2012, the US Food and Drug Administration approved the first subcutaneous ICD, which incorporates a generator and a lead that is implanted below the skin along the bottom of the rib cage and breast bone, removing the need for fluoroscopic guidance and direct vascular or cardiac access. Data in support of the approval were from a 33-center trial involving 321 patients who underwent ICD implantation or were undergoing replacement for a transvenous ICD.[178] A postmarket study will follow 1,616 patients for 5 years.

Evolution in programming algorithms may also alter the benefits harms balance.[179] As discussed above, MADIT-RIT showed mortality benefit for programming algorithms which may be additive to the benefit of an ICD alone.

Conclusions

There is a high strength of evidence that ICD therapy for primary prevention of SCD, versus no ICD therapy, shows benefit with regard to mortality and SCD in selected patients with reduced LVEF and ischemic or nonischemic cardiomyopathy. There is low strength of evidence that the risk of all-cause mortality is similar for patients who receive CRT-Ds versus ICD alone for primary prevention. A high strength of evidence shows overall early in-hospital adverse event rates of approximately 3 percent and serious adverse event rates of approximately 1 percent. Low strength of evidence shows variable late adverse events. Moderate strength of evidence shows inappropriate shocks are experienced by 3 to 21 percent of patients over 1 and 5 years of followup.

Acronyms

ADRIA	A+ versus DR Clinical Investigation of Arrhythmia Discrimination
AHRQ	Agency for Healthcare Research and Quality
AMIOVERT	Amiodarone Versus Implantable Cardioverter-Defibrillator: Randomized Trial in Patients With Nonischemic Dilated Cardiomyopathy and Asymptomatic Nonsustained Ventricular Tachycardia [trial]
AVID	Antiarrhythmics Versus Implantable Defibrillators [trial]
ATP	antitachycardia pacing
CABG	coronary artery bypass grafting
CABG-Patch	Coronary Artery Bypass Graft Patch [trial]
CAD	coronary artery disease
CAMIAT	Canadian Amiodarone Myocardial Infarction Arrhythmia Trial
CASH	Cardiac Arrest Study Hamburg
CAST	Cardiac Arrhythmia Suppression Trial
CAT	Cardiomyopathy Trial
CI	Confidence interval
CIDS	Canadian Implantable Defibrillator Study
CMS	Centers for Medicare and Medicaid Services
COMPANION	Comparison of Medical Therapy, Pacing and Defibrillation in Heart Failure [study]
CRT	cardiac resynchronization therapy
CRP-D	CRT with a biventricular defibrillator
CRT-P	CRT with a biventricular pacemaker (without a defibrillator)
DEFINITE	Defibrillators in Nonischemic Cardiomyopathy Treatment Evaluation
DINAMIT	Defibrillator in Acute Myocardial Infarction Trial
ECG	Electrocardiograms
EMIAT	European Myocardial Infarction Amiodarone Trial
ESRD	End stage renal disease
EPC	Evidence-based Practice Center
GWTG-HF	Get With the Guidelines-Heart Failure [study]
HR	hazard ratio
ICD	implantable cardioverter–defibrillator
IRIS	Immediate Risk Stratification Improves Survival [trial]
ITT	Intention-to-Treat
LV	left ventricular
LVEF	left ventricular ejection fraction
MADIT	Multicenter Automatic Defibrillator Implantation Trial
MADIT II	Multicenter Automatic Defibrillator Implantation Trial II
MADIT-CRT	Multicenter Automatic Defibrillator Implantation Trial with Cardiac Resynchronization Therapy
MENDMI	Prevention of Myocardial Enlargement and Dilation Post Myocardial Infarction [study]
MI	myocardial infarction
ms	millisecond(s)
NCDR	National Cardiovascular Data Registry
NNT	Number needed to treat
nRCS	nonrandomized comparative study
NYHA	New York Heart Association
OPTIMIZE-HF	Organized Program to Initiate Lifesaving Treatment in Hospitalized Patients with Heart Failure [study]
OR	odds ratio
QoL	quality of life
PCI	Percutaneous coronary intervention
RAFT	Resynchronization-Defibrillation for Ambulatory Heart Failure Trial

RCT	randomized controlled trial
RR	risk ratio
SA ECG	Signal Averaged ECG
SCD	sudden cardiac death
SCD-HeFT	Sudden Cardiac Death in Heart Failure Trial
SRDR	Systematic Review Data Repository
TOO	Task Order Officer
VF	ventricular fibrillation
VT	ventricular tachycardia

References

1. Adabag AS, Luepker RV, Roger VL, et al. Sudden cardiac death: epidemiology and risk factors. Nat Rev Cardiol 2010 Apr;7(4):216-25. PMID: *20142817*

2. Epstein, A. E., DiMarco, J. P., Ellenbogen, K. A., Estes, N. A., III, Freedman, R. A., Gettes, L. S et al. American College of Cardiology/American Heart Association Task Force on Practice Guidelines. Developed in collaboration with the American Association for Thoracic Surgery and Society of Thoracic Surgeons.[Erratum appears in Circulation.2009 Aug 4; 120(5):e34-5]. Circulation. 5-27-2008;117:e350-e408. *PMID: 18483207*

3. Lloyd-Jones, D., Adams, R. J., Brown, T. M., Carnethon, M., Dai, S., De, Simone G., Ferguson, T. B., et al. Executive summary: heart disease and stroke statistics--2010 update: a report from the American Heart Association.[Erratum appears in Circulation. 2010 Mar 30;121(12):e259]. Circulation. 2-23-2010;121:948-954. *PMID: 20177011*

4. Myerburg, R. J., Reddy, V., and Castellanos, A. Indications for implantable cardioverter-defibrillators based on evidence and judgment. J Am Coll Cardiol. 8-25-2009;54:747-763. *PMID: 19695452*

5. Rea, T. D. and Page, R. L. Community approaches to improve resuscitation after out-of-hospital sudden cardiac arrest. Circulation. 3-9-2010;121:1134-1140. *PMID: 20212292*

6. Zipes, D. P., Camm, A. J., Borggrefe, M., Buxton, A. E., Chaitman, B., Fromer, M., Gregoratos, G., et al. ACC/AHA/ESC 2006 Guidelines for Management of Patients With Ventricular Arrhythmias and the Prevention of Sudden Cardiac Death: a report of the American College of Cardiology/American Heart Association Task Force and the European Society of Cardiology Committee for Practice Guidelines: developed in collaboration with the European Heart Rhythm Association and the Heart Rhythm Society. Circulation. 9-5-2006;114:e385-e484. *PMID: 16935995*

7. American Heart Association: 2001 Heart and Stroke Statistical Update. 2000

8. Epstein, FH and Pisa, Z. International comparisons in ischemic heart disease mortality. Proc.Conf.Decline in Coronary Heart DiseaseMortality.DHEW, NIH Publication No.79-1610.U.S.Government. 197958-88.

9. Escobedo, L. G. and Zack, M. M. Comparison of sudden and nonsudden coronary deaths in the United States. Circulation. 6-1-1996;93:2033-2036. *PMID: 8640979*

10. Zheng, Z. J., Croft, J. B., Giles, W. H., and Mensah, G. A. Sudden cardiac death in the United States, 1989 to 1998. Circulation. 10-30-2001;104:2158-2163. *PMID: 11684624*

11. Deo, R. and Albert, C. M. Epidemiology and genetics of sudden cardiac death. Circulation. 1-31-2012;125:620-637. *PMID: 22294707*

12. Kuller, L., Lilienfeld, A., and Fisher, R. An epidemiological study of sudden and unexpected deaths in adults. Medicine (Baltimore). 1967;46:341-361. *PMID: 6043997*

13. Luu, M., Stevenson, W. G., Stevenson, L. W., Baron, K., and Walden, J. Diverse mechanisms of unexpected cardiac arrest in advanced heart failure. Circulation. 1989;80:1675-1680. *PMID: 2598430*

14. Myerburg, R. J., Kessler, K. M., and Castellanos, A. Sudden cardiac death. Structure, function, and time-dependence of risk. Circulation. 1992;85:Suppl-10. *PMID: 1728501*

15. Zipes, D. P. and Wellens, H. J. Sudden cardiac death. Circulation. 11-24-1998;98:2334-2351. *PMID: 9826323*

16. Survivors of out-of-hospital cardiac arrest with apparently normal heart. Need for definition and standardized clinical evaluation. Consensus Statement of the Joint Steering Committees of the Unexplained Cardiac Arrest Registry of Europe and of the Idiopathic Ventricular Fibrillation Registry of the United States. Circulation. 1997;95:265-272. *PMID: 8994445*

17. Fairbanks, R. J., Shah, M. N., Lerner, E. B., Ilangovan, K., Pennington, E. C., and Schneider, S. M. Epidemiology and outcomes of out-of-hospital cardiac arrest in Rochester, New York. Resuscitation. 2007;72:415-424. *PMID: 17174021*

18. Nichol, G., Thomas, E., Callaway, C. W., Hedges, J., Powell, J. L., Aufderheide, T. P., Rea, T., Lowe, R., Brown, T., Dreyer, J., Davis, D., Idris, A., Stiell, I., and Resuscitation Outcomes Consortium. Regional variation in out-of-hospital cardiac arrest incidence and outcome.[Erratum appears in JAMA. 2008 Oct 15;300(15):1763]. JAMA. 9-24-2008;300:1423-1431. *PMID: 18812533*

19. Fox, C. S., Evans, J. C., Larson, M. G., Lloyd-Jones, D. M., O'Donnell, C. J., Sorlie, P. D., Manolio, T. A., Kannel, W. B., and Levy, D. A comparison of death certificate out-of-hospital coronary heart disease death with physician-adjudicated sudden cardiac death. Am.J Cardiol. 4-1-2005;95:856-859. *PMID: 15781015*

20. Hinkle, L. E., Jr. and Thaler, H. T. Clinical classification of cardiac deaths. Circulation. 1982;65:457-464. *PMID: 7055867*

21. Connolly, S. J., Gent, M., Roberts, R. S., Dorian, P., Roy, D., Sheldon, R. S., Mitchell, L. B., Green, M. S., Klein, G. J., and O'Brien, B. Canadian implantable defibrillator study (CIDS) : a randomized trial of the implantable cardioverter defibrillator against amiodarone. Circulation. 3-21-2000;101:1297-1302. *PMID: 10725290*

22. Cairns, J. A., Connolly, S. J., Roberts, R., and Gent, M. Randomised trial of outcome after myocardial infarction in patients with frequent or repetitive ventricular premature depolarisations: CAMIAT. Canadian Amiodarone Myocardial Infarction Arrhythmia Trial Investigators.[Erratum appears in Lancet 1997 Jun 14;349(9067):1776]. Lancet. 3-8-1997;349:675-682. *PMID: 9078198*

23. Goldberger, J. J., Buxton, A. E., Cain, M., Costantini, O., Exner, D. V., Knight, B. P., Lloyd-Jones, D., Kadish, A. H., Lee, B., Moss, A., Myerburg, R., Olgin, J., Passman, R., Rosenbaum, D., Stevenson, W., Zareba, W., and Zipes, D. P. Risk stratification for arrhythmic sudden cardiac death: identifying the roadblocks. Circulation. 5-31-2011;123:2423-2430. *PMID: 21632516*

24. Lloyd-Jones, D. M., Hong, Y., Labarthe, D., Mozaffarian, D., Appel, L. J., Van, Horn L., Greenlund, K., et al. Defining and setting national goals for cardiovascular health promotion and disease reduction: the American Heart Association's strategic Impact Goal through 2020 and beyond. Circulation. 2-2-2010;121:586-613. *PMID: 20089546*

25. Holmberg, M., Holmberg, S., and Herlitz, J. Incidence, duration and survival of ventricular fibrillation in out-of-hospital cardiac arrest patients in sweden. Resuscitation. 2000;44:7-17. *PMID: 10699695*

26. Kuisma, M., Suominen, P., and Korpela, R. Paediatric out-of-hospital cardiac arrests-- epidemiology and outcome. Resuscitation. 1995;30:141-150. *PMID: 8560103*

27. Steinberger, J., Lucas, R. V., Jr., Edwards, J. E., and Titus, J. L. Causes of sudden unexpected cardiac death in the first two decades of life. Am.J Cardiol. 5-1-1996;77:992-995. *PMID: 8644651*

28. Wren, C., O'Sullivan, J. J., and Wright, C. Sudden death in children and adolescents. Heart. 2000;83:410-413. *PMID: 10722539*

29. Solomon, S. D., Zelenkofske, S., McMurray, J. J., Finn, P. V., Velazquez, E., Ertl, G., Harsanyi, A., Rouleau, J. L., Maggioni, A., Kober, L., White, H., Van de Werf, F., Pieper, K., Califf, R. M., Pfeffer, M. A., and Valsartan in Acute Myocardial Infarction Trial (VALIANT) Investigators. Sudden death in patients with myocardial infarction and left ventricular dysfunction, heart failure, or both.[Erratum appears in N Engl J Med. 2005 Aug 18;353(7):744]. New England Journal of Medicine. 6-23-2005;352:2581-2588. *PMID: 15972864*

30. Hallstrom, A. P., Cobb, L. A., and Ray, R. Smoking as a risk factor for recurrence of sudden cardiac arrest. N.Engl.J Med. 1-30-1986;314:271-275. *PMID: 3941718*

31. Cupples, L. A., Gagnon, D. R., and Kannel, W. B. Long- and short-term risk of sudden coronary death. Circulation. 1992;85:Suppl-8. *PMID: 1370216*

32. Jouven, X., Zureik, M., Desnos, M., Guerot, C., and Ducimetiere, P. Resting heart rate as a predictive risk factor for sudden death in middle-aged men. Cardiovasc Res. 2001;50:373-378. *PMID: 11334841*

33. Teodorescu, C., Reinier, K., Uy-Evanado, A., Navarro, J., Mariani, R., Gunson, K., Jui, J., and Chugh, S. S. Prolonged QRS duration on the resting ECG is associated with sudden death risk in coronary disease, independent of prolonged ventricular repolarization. Heart Rhythm. 2011;8:1562-1567. *PMID: 21699869*

34. Morin, D. P., Oikarinen, L., Viitasalo, M., Toivonen, L., Nieminen, M. S., Kjeldsen, S. E., Dahlof, B., John, M., Devereux, R. B., and Okin, P. M. QRS duration predicts sudden cardiac death in hypertensive patients undergoing intensive medical therapy: the LIFE study. Eur Heart J. 2009;30:2908-2914. *PMID: 19687165*

35. Algra, A., Tijssen, J. G., Roelandt, J. R., Pool, J., and Lubsen, J. QTc prolongation measured by standard 12-lead electrocardiography is an independent risk factor for sudden death due to cardiac arrest. Circulation. 1991;83:1888-1894. *PMID: 2040041*

36. Straus, S. M., Kors, J. A., De Bruin, M. L., van der Hooft, C. S., Hofman, A., Heeringa, J., Deckers, J. W., Kingma, J. H., Sturkenboom, M. C., Stricker, B. H., and Witteman, J. C. Prolonged QTc interval and risk of sudden cardiac death in a population of older adults. J Am Coll Cardiol. 1-17-2006;47:362-367. *PMID: 16412861*

37. Passman, R. and Goldberger, J. J. Predicting the future: risk stratification for sudden cardiac death in patients with left ventricular dysfunction. Circulation. 6-19-2012;125:3031-3037. *PMID: 22711668*

38. Stecker, E. C., Vickers, C., Waltz, J., Socoteanu, C., John, B. T., Mariani, R., McAnulty, J. H., Gunson, K., Jui, J., and Chugh, S. S. Population-based analysis of sudden cardiac death with and without left ventricular systolic dysfunction: two-year findings from the Oregon Sudden Unexpected Death Study. J Am.Coll.Cardiol. 3-21-2006;47:1161-1166. *PMID: 16545646*

39. Atwater, B. D., Thompson, V. P., Vest, R. N., III, Shaw, L. K., Mazzei, W. R., Jr., Al-Khatib, S. M., Hranitzky, P. M., Bahnson, T. D., Velazquez, E. J., Califf, R. M., Lee, K. L., and Roe, M. T. Usefulness of the Duke Sudden Cardiac Death risk score for predicting sudden cardiac death in patients with angiographic (>75% narrowing) coronary artery disease. Am.J Cardiol. 12-15-2009;104:1624-1630. *PMID: 19962465*

40. Goldenberg, I., Vyas, A. K., Hall, W. J., Moss, A. J., Wang, H., He, H., Zareba, W., McNitt, S., and Andrews, M. L. Risk stratification for primary implantation of a cardioverter-defibrillator in patients with ischemic left ventricular dysfunction. J Am.Coll.Cardiol. 1-22-2008;51:288-296. *PMID: 18206738*

41. Buxton, A. E., Lee, K. L., DiCarlo, L., Gold, M. R., Greer, G. S., Prystowsky, F. N., O'Toole, M. F., Tang, A., Fisher, J. D., Coromilas, J., Talajic, M., and Hafley, G. Electrophysiologic testing to identify patients with coronary artery disease who are at risk for sudden death. Multicenter Unsustained Tachycardia Trial Investigators. N.Engl.J.Med. 6-29-2000;342:1937-1945. *PMID: 10874061*

42. Moss, A. J., Hall, W. J., Cannom, D. S., Daubert, J. P., Higgins, S. L., Klein, H., Levine, J. H., Saksena, S., Waldo, A. L., Wilber, D., Brown, M. W., and Heo, M. Improved survival with an implanted defibrillator in patients with coronary disease at high risk for ventricular arrhythmia. Multicenter Automatic Defibrillator Implantation Trial Investigators. N.Engl.J.Med. 12-26-1996;335:1933-1940. *PMID: 8960472*

43. Adabag, A. S., Therneau, T. M., Gersh, B. J., Weston, S. A., and Roger, V. L. Sudden death after myocardial infarction. JAMA. 11-5-2008;300:2022-2029. *PMID: 18984889*

44. Preliminary report: effect of encainide and flecainide on mortality in a randomized trial of arrhythmia suppression after myocardial infarction. The Cardiac Arrhythmia Suppression Trial (CAST) Investigators. New England Journal of Medicine. 8-10-1989;321:406-412. *PMID: 2473403*

45. Effect of the antiarrhythmic agent moricizine on survival after myocardial infarction. The Cardiac Arrhythmia Suppression Trial II Investigators. New England Journal of Medicine. 7-23-1992;327:227-233. *PMID: 1377359*

46. Waldo, A. L., Camm, A. J., deRuyter, H., Friedman, P. L., MacNeil, D. J., Pauls, J. F., Pitt, B., Pratt, C. M., Schwartz, P. J., and Veltri, E. P. Effect of d-sotalol on mortality in patients with left ventricular dysfunction after recent and remote myocardial infarction. The SWORD Investigators. Survival With Oral d-Sotalol.[Erratum appears in Lancet 1996 Aug 10;348(9024):416]. Lancet. 7-6-1996;348:7-12. *PMID: 8691967*

47. Christiansen, C. B., Torp-Pedersen, C., and Kober, L. Impact of dronedarone in atrial fibrillation and flutter on stroke reduction. Clin Interv Aging. 2010;5:63-69. *PMID: 20396635*

48. Camm, A. J., Julian, D., Janse, G., Munoz, A., Schwartz, P., Simon, P., and Frangin, G. The European Myocardial Infarct Amiodarone Trial (EMIAT). EMIAT Investigators. Am J Cardiol. 11-26-1993;72:95F-98F. *PMID: 8237837*

49. Kuck, K. H., Cappato, R., Siebels, J., and Ruppel, R. Randomized comparison of antiarrhythmic drug therapy with implantable defibrillators in patients resuscitated from cardiac arrest : the Cardiac Arrest Study Hamburg (CASH). Circulation. 8-15-2000;102:748-754. *PMID: 10942742*

50. Causes of death in the Antiarrhythmics Versus Implantable Defibrillators (AVID) Trial. J Am Coll Cardiol. 11-1-1999;34:1552-1559. *PMID: 10551706*

51. Bardy, G. H., Lee, K. L., Mark, D. B., Poole, J. E., Packer, D. L., Boineau, R., Domanski, M., Troutman, C., Anderson, J., Johnson, G., McNulty, S. E., Clapp-Channing, N., vidson-Ray, L. D., Fraulo, E. S., Fishbein, D. P., Luceri, R. M., and Ip, J. H. Amiodarone or an implantable cardioverter-defibrillator for congestive heart failure. N.Engl.J.Med. 1-20-2005;352:225-237. *PMID: 15659722*

52. Mirowski, M., Reid, P. R., Mower, M. M., Watkins, L., Gott, V. L., Schauble, J. F., Langer, A., Heilman, M. S., Kolenik, S. A., Fischell, R. E., and Weisfeldt, M. L. Termination of malignant ventricular arrhythmias with an implanted automatic defibrillator in human beings. New England Journal of Medicine. 8-7-1980;303:322-324. *PMID: 6991948*

53. Carroll, D. L. and Hamilton, G. A. Quality of life in implanted cardioverter defibrillator recipients: the impact of a device shock. Heart Lung. 2005;34:169-178. *PMID: 16015221*

54. Irvine, J., Dorian, P., Baker, B., O'Brien, B. J., Roberts, R., Gent, M., Newman, D., and Connolly, S. J. Quality of life in the Canadian Implantable Defibrillator Study (CIDS). Am Heart J. 2002;144:282-289. *PMID: 12177646*

55. Schron, E. B., Exner, D. V., Yao, Q., Jenkins, L. S., Steinberg, J. S., Cook, J. R., Kutalek, S. P., Friedman, P. L., Bubien, R. S., Page, R. L., and Powell, J. Quality of life in the antiarrhythmics versus implantable defibrillators trial: impact of therapy and influence of adverse symptoms and defibrillator shocks. Circulation. 2-5-2002;105:589-594. *PMID: 11827924*

56. Grimm, W., Plachta, E., and Maisch, B. Antitachycardia pacing for spontaneous rapid ventricular tachycardia in patients with prophylactic cardioverter-defibrillator therapy. Pacing Clin Electrophysiol. 2006;29:759-764. *PMID: 16884513*

57. Wathen, M. S., DeGroot, P. J., Sweeney, M. O., Stark, A. J., Otterness, M. F., Adkisson, W. O., Canby, R. C., Khalighi, K., Machado, C., Rubenstein, D. S., Volosin, K. J., and PainFREE Rx, I. I. I. Prospective randomized multicenter trial of empirical antitachycardia pacing versus shocks for spontaneous rapid ventricular tachycardia in patients with implantable cardioverter-defibrillators: Pacing Fast Ventricular Tachycardia Reduces Shock Therapies (PainFREE Rx II) trial results. Circulation. 10-26-2004;110:2591-2596. *PMID: 15492306*

58. Wilkoff, B. L., Ousdigian, K. T., Sterns, L. D., Wang, Z. J., Wilson, R. D., Morgan, J. M., and EMPIRIC, Trial, I. A comparison of empiric to physician-tailored programming of implantable cardioverter-defibrillators: results from the prospective randomized multicenter EMPIRIC trial. J Am Coll Cardiol. 7-18-2006;48:330-339. *PMID: 16843184*

59. Wilkoff, B. L., Williamson, B. D., Stern, R. S., Moore, S. L., Lu, F., Lee, S. W., Birgersdotter-Green, U. M., Wathen, M. S., Van Gelder, I. C., Heubner, B. M., Brown, M. L., Holloman, K. K., and PREPARE, Study, I. Strategic programming of detection and therapy parameters in implantable cardioverter-defibrillators reduces shocks in primary prevention patients: results from the PREPARE (Primary Prevention Parameters Evaluation) study. J Am Coll Cardiol. 8-12-2008;52:541-550. *PMID: 18687248*

60. Moss, A. J., Schuger, C., Beck, C. A., Brown, M. W., Cannom, D. S., Daubert, J. P., Estes, N. A., III, Greenberg, H., Hall, W. J., Huang, D. T., Kautzner, J., Klein, H., McNitt, S., Olshansky, B., Shoda, M., Wilber, D., and Zareba, W. Reduction in Inappropriate Therapy and Mortality through ICD Programming. N.Engl.J.Med. 11-6-2012 *PMID: 23131066*

61. Bernard, M. L., Shotwell, M., Nietert, P. J., and Gold, M. R. Meta-analysis of bleeding complications associated with cardiac rhythm device implantation. Circ.Arrhythm.Electrophysiol. 6-1-2012;5:468-474. *PMID: 22554249*

62. Cheng, A., Wang, Y., Curtis, J. P., and Varosy, P. D. Acute lead dislodgements and in-hospital mortality in patients enrolled in the national cardiovascular data registry implantable cardioverter defibrillator registry. J.Am.Coll.Cardiol. 11-9-2010;56:1651-1656. *PMID: 21050975*

63. Polin, G. M., Zado, E., Nayak, H., Cooper, J. M., Russo, A. M., Dixit, S., Lin, D., Marchlinski, F. E., and Verdino, R. J. Proper management of pericardial tamponade as a late complication of implantable cardiac device placement. Am.J Cardiol. 7-15-2006;98:223-225. *PMID: 16828597*

64. Sohail, M. R., Henrikson, C. A., Braid-Forbes, M. J., Forbes, K. F., and Lerner, D. J. Mortality and cost associated with cardiovascular implantable electronic device infections. Arch.Intern.Med. 11-14-2011;171:1821-1828. *PMID: 21911623*

65. van Rees, J. B., de Bie, M. K., Thijssen, J., Borleffs, C. J., Schalij, M. J., and van, Erven L. Implantation-related complications of implantable cardioverter-defibrillators and cardiac resynchronization therapy devices: a systematic review of randomized clinical trials. J Am.Coll.Cardiol. 8-30-2011;58:995-1000. *PMID: 21867832*

66. Curtis, J. P., Luebbert, J. J., Wang, Y., Rathore, S. S., Chen, J., Heidenreich, P. A., Hammill, S. C., Lampert, R. I., and Krumholz, H. M. Association of physician certification and outcomes among patients receiving an implantable cardioverter-defibrillator. JAMA. 4-22-2009;301:1661-1670. *PMID: 19383957*

67. Freeman, J. V., Wang, Y., Curtis, J. P., Heidenreich, P. A., and Hlatky, M. A. Physician procedure volume and complications of cardioverter-defibrillator implantation. Circulation. 1-3-2012;125:57-64. *PMID: 22095828*

68. Berdowski, J., ten, Haaf M., Tijssen, J. G., Chapman, F. W., and Koster, R. W. Time in recurrent ventricular fibrillation and survival after out-of-hospital cardiac arrest. Circulation. 9-14-2010;122:1101-1108. *PMID: 20805427*

69. Epstein, A. E., DiMarco, J. P., Ellenbogen, K. A., Estes, N. A., III, Freedman, R. A., Gettes, L. S., Gillinov, A. M., et al. ACC/AHA/HRS 2008 Guidelines for Device-Based Therapy of Cardiac Rhythm Abnormalities: a report of the American College of Cardiology/American Heart Association Task Force on Practice Guidelines developed in collaboration with the American Association for Thoracic Surgery and Society of Thoracic Surgeons.[Erratum appears in J Am Coll Cardiol. 2009 Apr 21;53(16):1473], [Erratum appears in J Am Coll Cardiol. 2009 Jan 6;53(1):147]. J Am Coll Cardiol. 5-27-2008;51:e1-62. *PMID: 18498951*

70. Gregoratos, G., Abrams, J., Epstein, A. E., Freedman, R. A., Hayes, D. L., Hlatky, M. A., Kerber, R. E., Naccarelli, G. V., Schoenfeld, M. H., Silka, M. J., and Winters, S. L. ACC/AHA/NASPE 2002 Guideline Update for Implantation of Cardiac Pacemakers and Antiarrhythmia Devices--summary article: a report of the American College of Cardiology/American Heart Association Task Force on Practice Guidelines (ACC/AHA/NASPE Committee to Update the 1998 Pacemaker Guidelines). J Am Coll Cardiol. 11-6-2002;40:1703-1719. *PMID: 12427427*

71. Tracy, C. M., Epstein, A. E., Darbar, D., DiMarco, J. P., Dunbar, S. B., Estes, N. A., III, Ferguson, T. B., Jr., Hammill, S. C., Karasik, P. E., Link, M. S., Marine, J. E., Schoenfeld, M. H., Shanker, A. J., Silka, M. J., Stevenson, L. W., Stevenson, W. G., and Varosy, P. D. 2012 ACCF/AHA/HRS Focused Update of the 2008 Guidelines for

Device-Based Therapy of Cardiac Rhythm Abnormalities: A Report of the American College of Cardiology Foundation/American Heart Association Task Force on Practice Guidelines. J Am Coll Cardiol. 10-2-2012;60:1297-1313. *PMID: 22975230*

72. Linde, C., Abraham, W. T., Gold, M. R., St John, Sutton M., Ghio, S., Daubert, C., and REVERSE (REsynchronization reVErses Remodeling in Systolic left vEntricular dysfunction) Study Group. Randomized trial of cardiac resynchronization in mildly symptomatic heart failure patients and in asymptomatic patients with left ventricular dysfunction and previous heart failure symptoms. J Am Coll Cardiol. 12-2-2008;52:1834-1843. *PMID: 19038680*

73. Moss, Arthur J., Hall, W. Jackson, Cannom, David S., Klein, Helmut, Brown, Mary W., Daubert, James P., Estes, N. A. M., Foster, Elyse, Greenberg, Henry, Higgins, Steven L., Pfeffer, Marc A., Solomon, Scott D., Wilber, David, and Zareba, Wojciech. Cardiac-Resynchronization Therapy for the Prevention of Heart-Failure Events. New England Journal of Medicine. 10-1-2009;361:1329-1338.

74. Tang, A. S., Wells, G. A., Talajic, M., Arnold, M. O., Sheldon, R., Connolly, S., Hohnloser, S. H., Nichol, G., Birnie, D. H., Sapp, J. L., Yee, R., Healey, J. S., Rouleau, J. L., and Resynchronization-Defibrillation for Ambulatory Heart Failure Trial Investigators. Cardiac-resynchronization therapy for mild-to-moderate heart failure. New England Journal of Medicine. 12-16-2010;363:2385-2395. *PMID: 21073365*

75. Russo, A. M., Stainback, R. F., Bailey, S. R., Epstein, A. E., Heidenreich, P. A., Jessup, M., Kapa, S., Kremers, M. S., Lindsay, B. D., and Stevenson, L. W. ACCF/HRS/AHA/ASE/HFSA/SCAI/SCCT/SCMR 2013 appropriate use criteria for implantable cardioverter-defibrillators and cardiac resynchronization therapy: a report of the American College of Cardiology Foundation appropriate use criteria task force, Heart Rhythm Society, American Heart Association, American Society of Echocardiography, Heart Failure Society of America, Society for Cardiovascular Angiography and Interventions, Society of Cardiovascular Computed Tomography, and Society for Cardiovascular Magnetic Resonance. Heart Rhythm. 2013;10:e11-e58. *PMID: 23473952*

76. Moss, A. J., Zareba, W., Hall, W. J., Klein, H., Wilber, D. J., Cannom, D. S., Daubert, J. P., Higgins, S. L., Brown, M. W., Andrews, M. L., and Multicenter Automatic Defibrillator Implantation Trial II investigators. Prophylactic implantation of a defibrillator in patients with myocardial infarction and reduced ejection fraction. New England Journal of Medicine. 3-21-2002;346:877-883. *PMID: 11907286*

77. Decision Memo for Implantable Defibrillators (CAG-00157R3), http://www.cms.gov/medicare-coverage-database/details/nca-decision-memo.aspx?NCAId=148&NCDId=110&ncdver=3&NcaName=Implantable+Defibrillators&IsPopup=y&bc=AAAAAAAAEAAA&, last accessed 1/8/13. 2005

78. Agency for Healthcare Research and Quality. Methods Guide for Effectiveness and Comparative Effectiveness Reviews. AHRQ. 2011;AHRQ Publication No. 10(11)-EHC063-

EF.:*http://www.effectivehealthcare.ahrq.gov/ehc/products/60/318/MethodsGuide_Prepub lication_Draft_20110824.pdf*

79. Hammill, S. C., Kremers, M. S., Kadish, A. H., Stevenson, L. W., Heidenreich, P. A., Lindsay, B. D., Mirro, M. J., Radford, M. J., McKay, C., Wang, Y., Lang, C. M., Pontzer, K., Rumsfeld, J., Phurrough, S. E., Curtis, J. P., and Brindis, R. G. Review of the ICD Registry's third year, expansion to include lead data and pediatric ICD procedures, and role for measuring performance. Heart Rhythm. 2009;6:1397-1401. *PMID: 19716099*

80. Wallace, B. C., Trikalinos, T. A., Lau, J., Brodley, C., and Schmid, C. H. Semi-automated screening of biomedical citations for systematic reviews. BMC Bioinform. 2010;11:55. *PMID: 20102628*

81. Lau, J. Proposed Governance and Data Management Policy for the Systematic Review Data Repository. Agency for Healthcare Research and Quality. 2012

82. Higgins J.P. Cochrane handbook for systematic reviews of interventions. Version 5.0.2. [updated September 2009]. The Cochrane Collaboration. 2009

83. Chou, R., Aronson, N., Atkins, D., Ismaila, A. S., Santaguida, P., Smith, D. H., Whitlock, E., Wilt, T. J., and Moher, D. AHRQ series paper 4: assessing harms when comparing medical interventions: AHRQ and the effective health-care program. J.Clin.Epidemiol. 2010;63:502-512. *PMID: 18823754*

84. Santaguida, P, Raina, P, and Ismaila, A. McMaster Quality Assessment Scale of Harms (McHarm) for primary studies, http://bmg.cochrane.org/sites/bmg.cochrane.org/files/uploads/McHarm%20for%20Primary%20Studies.pdf, last accessed 1/8/13.

85. DerSimonian, R. and Laird, N. Meta-analysis in clinical trials. Control Clin.Trials. 1986;7:177-188. *PMID: 3802833*

86. Tierney, J. F., Stewart, L. A., Ghersi, D, Burdett, S, and Sydes, M. R. Practical methods for incorporating summary time-to-event data into meta-analysis. Trials. 2007;8:16. *PMID:*

87. Higgins, J. P. and Thompson, S. G. Quantifying heterogeneity in a meta-analysis. Stat.Med. 6-15-2002;21:1539-1558. *PMID: 12111919*

88. Higgins, J. P., Thompson, S. G., Deeks, J. J., and Altman, D. G. Measuring inconsistency in meta-analyses. BMJ. 9-6-2003;327:557-560. *PMID: 12958120*

89. Altman, D. G. and Andersen, P. K. Calculating the number needed to treat for trials where the outcome is time to an event. BMJ. 12-4-1999;319:1492-1495. *PMID: 10582940*

90. Owens, D. K., Lohr, K. N., Atkins, D., Treadwell, J. R., Reston, J. T., Bass, E. B., Chang, S., and Helfand, M. AHRQ series paper 5: grading the strength of a body of evidence

when comparing medical interventions--agency for healthcare research and quality and the effective health-care program. Journal of Clinical Epidemiology. 2010;63:513-523. *PMID: 19595577*

91. Bansch, D., Antz, M., Boczor, S., Volkmer, M., Tebbenjohanns, J., Seidl, K., Block, M., Gietzen, F., Berger, J., and Kuck, K. H. Primary prevention of sudden cardiac death in idiopathic dilated cardiomyopathy: the Cardiomyopathy Trial (CAT). Circulation. 3-26-2002;105:1453-1458. *PMID: 11914254*

92. Barsheshet, A., Moss, A. J., McNitt, S., Jons, C., Glikson, M., Klein, H. U., Huang, D. T., Steinberg, J. S., Brown, M. W., Zareba, W., and Goldenberg, I. Long-term implications of cumulative right ventricular pacing among patients with an implantable cardioverter-defibrillator. Heart Rhythm. 2011;8:212-218. *PMID: 21044897*

93. Berenbom, L. D., Weiford, B. C., Vacek, J. L., Emert, M. P., Hall, W. J., Andrews, M. L., McNitt, S., Zareba, W., and Moss, A. J. Differences in outcomes between patients treated with single- versus dual-chamber implantable cardioverter defibrillators: a substudy of the Multicenter Automatic Defibrillator Implantation Trial II. Ann.Noninvasive.Electrocardiol. 2005;10:429-435. *PMID: 16255753*

94. Bigger, J. T., Jr. Prophylactic use of implanted cardiac defibrillators in patients at high risk for ventricular arrhythmias after coronary-artery bypass graft surgery. Coronary Artery Bypass Graft (CABG) Patch Trial Investigators. N.Engl.J.Med. 11-27-1997;337:1569-1575. *PMID: 9371853*

95. Bristow, M. R., Saxon, L. A., Boehmer, J., Krueger, S., Kass, D. A., De, Marco T., Carson, P., DiCarlo, L., DeMets, D., White, B. G., DeVries, D. W., and Feldman, A. M. Cardiac-resynchronization therapy with or without an implantable defibrillator in advanced chronic heart failure. N.Engl.J.Med. 5-20-2004;350:2140-2150. *PMID: 15152059*

96. Goldenberg, I., Moss, A. J., McNitt, S., Zareba, W., Hall, W. J., Andrews, M. L., Wilber, D. J., and Klein, H. U. Time dependence of defibrillator benefit after coronary revascularization in the Multicenter Automatic Defibrillator Implantation Trial (MADIT)-II. J.Am.Coll.Cardiol. 5-2-2006;47:1811-1817. *PMID: 16682305*

97. Goldenberg, I., Moss, A. J., McNitt, S., Zareba, W., Andrews, M. L., Hall, W. J., Greenberg, H., and Case, R. B. Relations among renal function, risk of sudden cardiac death, and benefit of the implanted cardiac defibrillator in patients with ischemic left ventricular dysfunction. Am.J.Cardiol. 8-15-2006;98:485-490. *PMID: 16893702*

98. Hohnloser, S. H., Kuck, K. H., Dorian, P., Roberts, R. S., Hampton, J. R., Hatala, R., Fain, E., Gent, M., and Connolly, S. J. Prophylactic use of an implantable cardioverter-defibrillator after acute myocardial infarction. N.Engl.J.Med. 12-9-2004;351:2481-2488. *PMID: 15590950*

99. Kadish, A., Dyer, A., Daubert, J. P., Quigg, R., Estes, N. A., Anderson, K. P., Calkins, H., Hoch, D., Goldberger, J., Shalaby, A., Sanders, W. E., Schaechter, A., and Levine, J.

H. Prophylactic defibrillator implantation in patients with nonischemic dilated cardiomyopathy. N.Engl.J.Med. 5-20-2004;350:2151-2158. *PMID: 15152060*

100. Namerow, P. B., Firth, B. R., Heywood, G. M., Windle, J. R., and Parides, M. K. Quality-of-life six months after CABG surgery in patients randomized to ICD versus no ICD therapy: findings from the CABG Patch Trial. Pacing Clin.Electrophysiol. 1999;22:1305-1313. *PMID: 10527011*

101. Noyes, K., Corona, E., Zwanziger, J., Hall, W. J., Zhao, H., Wang, H., Moss, A. J., and Dick, A. W. Health-related quality of life consequences of implantable cardioverter defibrillators: results from MADIT II. Med.Care. 2007;45:377-385. *PMID: 17446823*

102. Steinbeck, G., Andresen, D., Seidl, K., Brachmann, J., Hoffmann, E., Wojciechowski, D., Kornacewicz-Jach, Z., Sredniawa, B., Lupkovics, G., Hofgartner, F., Lubinski, A., Rosenqvist, M., Habets, A., Wegscheider, K., and Senges, J. Defibrillator implantation early after myocardial infarction. N.Engl.J.Med. 10-8-2009;361:1427-1436. *PMID: 19812399*

103. Strickberger, S. A., Hummel, J. D., Bartlett, T. G., Frumin, H. I., Schuger, C. D., Beau, S. L., Bitar, C., and Morady, F. Amiodarone versus implantable cardioverter-defibrillator:randomized trial in patients with nonischemic dilated cardiomyopathy and asymptomatic nonsustained ventricular tachycardia--AMIOVIRT. J.Am.Coll.Cardiol. 5-21-2003;41:1707-1712. *PMID: 12767651*

104. Wilber, D. J., Zareba, W., Hall, W. J., Brown, M. W., Lin, A. C., Andrews, M. L., Burke, M., and Moss, A. J. Time dependence of mortality risk and defibrillator benefit after myocardial infarction. Circulation. 3-9-2004;109:1082-1084. *PMID: 14993128*

105. Chan, P. S., Nallamothu, B. K., Spertus, J. A., Masoudi, F. A., Bartone, C., Kereiakes, D. J., and Chow, T. Impact of age and medical comorbidity on the effectiveness of implantable cardioverter-defibrillators for primary prevention. Circ.Cardiovasc.Qual.Outcomes. 2009;2:16-24. *PMID: 20031808*

106. Fonarow, G. C., Feliciano, Z., Boyle, N. G., Knight, L., Woo, M. A., Moriguchi, J. D., Laks, H., and Wiener, I. Improved survival in patients with nonischemic advanced heart failure and syncope treated with an implantable cardioverter-defibrillator. Am.J.Cardiol. 4-15-2000;85:981-985. *PMID: 10760339*

107. Hernandez, A. F., Fonarow, G. C., Hammill, B. G., Al-Khatib, S. M., Yancy, C. W., O'Connor, C. M., Schulman, K. A., Peterson, E. D., and Curtis, L. H. Clinical effectiveness of implantable cardioverter-defibrillators among medicare beneficiaries with heart failure. Circ.Heart Fail. 2010;3:7-13. *PMID: 20009044*

108. Mezu, U., Adelstein, E., Jain, S., and Saba, S. Effectiveness of implantable defibrillators in octogenarians and nonagenarians for primary prevention of sudden cardiac death. Am.J.Cardiol. 9-1-2011;108:718-722. *PMID: 21640321*

109. Al-Khatib, S. M., Hellkamp, A. S., Lee, K. L., Anderson, J., Poole, J. E., Mark, D. B., and Bardy, G. H. Implantable cardioverter defibrillator therapy in patients with prior coronary revascularization in the Sudden Cardiac Death in Heart Failure Trial (SCD-HeFT). J.Cardiovasc.Electrophysiol. 2008;19:1059-1065. *PMID: 18479330*

110. Piccini, J. P., Al-Khatib, S. M., Hellkamp, A. S., Anstrom, K. J., Poole, J. E., Mark, D. B., Lee, K. L., and Bardy, G. H. Mortality benefits from implantable cardioverter-defibrillator therapy are not restricted to patients with remote myocardial infarction: an analysis from the Sudden Cardiac Death in Heart Failure Trial (SCD-HeFT). Heart Rhythm. 2011;8:393-400. *PMID: 21109025*

111. Chung, E. S., Dan, D., Solomon, S. D., Bank, A. J., Pastore, J., Iyer, A., Berger, R. D., Franklin, J. O., Jones, G., Machado, C., and Stolen, C. M. Effect of peri-infarct pacing early after myocardial infarction: results of the prevention of myocardial enlargement and dilatation post myocardial infarction study. Circ.Heart Fail. 2010;3:650-658. *PMID: 20852059*

112. Diab, I. G., Hunter, R. J., Kamdar, R., Berriman, T., Duncan, E., Richmond, L., Baker, V., Abrams, D., Earley, M. J., Sporton, S., and Schilling, R. J. Does ventricular dyssynchrony on echocardiography predict response to cardiac resynchronisation therapy? A randomised controlled study. Heart. 2011;97:1410-1416. *PMID: 21700757*

113. Barsheshet, A., Goldenberg, I., Narins, C. R., Moss, A. J., McNitt, S., Wang, P. J., Huang, D. T., Hall, W. J., Zareba, W., Eldar, M., and Guetta, V. Time dependence of life-threatening ventricular tachyarrhythmias after coronary revascularization in MADIT-CRT. Heart Rhythm. 2010;7:1421-1427. *PMID: 20620231*

114. Aggarwal, A., Wang, Y., Rumsfeld, J. S., Curtis, J. P., and Heidenreich, P. A. Clinical characteristics and in-hospital outcome of patients with end-stage renal disease on dialysis referred for implantable cardioverter-defibrillator implantation. Heart Rhythm. 2009;6:1565-1571. *PMID: 19879533*

115. Dewland, T. A., Pellegrini, C. N., Wang, Y., Marcus, G. M., Keung, E., and Varosy, P. D. Dual-chamber implantable cardioverter-defibrillator selection is associated with increased complication rates and mortality among patients enrolled in the NCDR implantable cardioverter-defibrillator registry. J.Am.Coll.Cardiol. 8-30-2011;58:1007-1013. *PMID: 21867834*

116. Freeman, J. V., Wang, Y., Curtis, J. P., Heidenreich, P. A., and Hlatky, M. A. The relation between hospital procedure volume and complications of cardioverter-defibrillator implantation from the implantable cardioverter-defibrillator registry. J.Am.Coll.Cardiol. 9-28-2010;56:1133-1139. *PMID: 20863954*

117. Haines, D. E., Wang, Y., and Curtis, J. Implantable cardioverter-defibrillator registry risk score models for acute procedural complications or death after implantable cardioverter-defibrillator implantation. Circulation. 5-17-2011;123:2069-2076. *PMID: 21537001*

118. Peterson, P. N., Daugherty, S. L., Wang, Y., Vidaillet, H. J., Heidenreich, P. A., Curtis, J. P., and Masoudi, F. A. Gender differences in procedure-related adverse events in patients receiving implantable cardioverter-defibrillator therapy. Circulation. 3-3-2009;119:1078-1084. *PMID: 19221223*

119. Tsai, V., Goldstein, M. K., Hsia, H. H., Wang, Y., Curtis, J., and Heidenreich, P. A. Age differences in primary prevention implantable cardioverter-defibrillator use in U.S. individuals. J Am Geriatr Soc. 2011;59:1589-1595. *PMID: 21883101*

120. Tsai, V., Goldstein, M. K., Hsia, H. H., Wang, Y., Curtis, J., and Heidenreich, P. A. Influence of age on perioperative complications among patients undergoing implantable cardioverter-defibrillators for primary prevention in the United States. Circ Cardiovasc Qual Outcomes. 2011;4:549-556. *PMID: 21878667*

121. Wei, S., Loyo-Berrios, N. I., Haigney, M. C., Cheng, H., Pinnow, E. E., Mitchell, K. R., Beachy, J. H., Woodward, A. M., Wang, Y., Curtis, J. P., and Marinac-Dabic, D. Elevated B-type natriuretic peptide is associated with increased in-hospital mortality or cardiac arrest in patients undergoing implantable cardioverter-defibrillator implantation. Circ.Cardiovasc.Qual.Outcomes. 2011;4:346-354. *PMID: 21487093*

122. Sticherling, C., Zabel, M., Spencker, S., Meyerfeldt, U., Eckardt, L., Behrens, S., Niehaus, M., and ADRIA, Investigators. Comparison of a novel, single-lead atrial sensing system with a dual-chamber implantable cardioverter-defibrillator system in patients without antibradycardia pacing indications: results of a randomized study. Circ Arrhythm Electrophysiol. 2011;4:56-63. *PMID: 21156772*

123. Birnie, D. H., Parkash, R., Exner, D. V., Essebag, V., Healey, J. S., Verma, A., Coutu, B., Kus, T., Mangat, I., Ayala-Paredes, F., Nery, P., Wells, G., and Krahn, A. D. Clinical predictors of Fidelis lead failure: report from the Canadian Heart Rhythm Society Device Committee. Circulation. 3-13-2012;125:1217-1225. *PMID: 22311781*

124. Borleffs, C. J., van, Erven L., van Bommel, R. J., van der Velde, E. T., van der Wall, E. E., Bax, J. J., Rosendaal, F. R., and Schalij, M. J. Risk of failure of transvenous implantable cardioverter-defibrillator leads. Circ Arrhythm Electrophysiol. 2009;2:411-416. *PMID: 19808497*

125. Brullmann, S., Dichtl, W., Paoli, U., Haegeli, L., Schmied, C., Steffel, J., Brunckhorst, C., Hintringer, F., Seifert, B., Duru, F., and Wolber, T. Comparison of benefit and mortality of implantable cardioverter-defibrillator therapy in patients aged >=75 years versus those <75 years. Am J Cardiol. 3-1-2012;109:712-717. *PMID: 22154315*

126. Brumberg, G. E., Kaseer, B., Shah, H., Saba, S., and Jain, S. Biventricular defibrillator patients have higher complication rates after revision of recalled leads. Pacing Clin Electrophysiol. 2012;35:665-671. *PMID: 22519559*

127. Charytan, D. M., Patrick, A. R., Liu, J., Setoguchi, S., Herzog, C. A., Brookhart, M. A., and Winkelmayer, W. C. Trends in the use and outcomes of implantable cardioverter-

defibrillators in patients undergoing dialysis in the United States. Am J Kidney Dis. 2011;58:409-417. *PMID: 21664735*

128. de Bie, M. K., van Rees, J. B., Thijssen, J., Borleffs, C. J., Trines, S. A., Cannegieter, S. C., Schalij, M. J., and van, Erven L. Cardiac device infections are associated with a significant mortality risk. Heart Rhythm. 2012;9:494-498. *PMID: 22056722*

129. Dichtl, W., Wolber, T., Paoli, U., Brullmann, S., Stuhlinger, M., Berger, T., Spuller, K., Strasak, A., Pachinger, O., Haegeli, L. M., Duru, F., and Hintringer, F. Appropriate therapy but not inappropriate shocks predict survival in implantable cardioverter defibrillator patients. Clin Cardiol. 2011;34:433-436. *PMID: 21678454*

130. Gradaus, R., Block, M., Brachmann, J., Breithardt, G., Huber, H. G., Jung, W., Kranig, W., Mletzko, R. U., Schoels, W., Seidl, K., Senges, J., Siebels, J., Steinbeck, G., Stellbrink, C., Andresen, D., and German, EURID Registry. Mortality, morbidity, and complications in 3344 patients with implantable cardioverter defibrillators: results fron the German ICD Registry EURID. Pacing Clin Electrophysiol. 2003;26:t-8. *PMID: 12914630*

131. Hauser, R. G., Mugglin, A. S., Friedman, P. A., Kramer, D. B., Kallinen, L., McGriff, D., and Hayes, D. L. Early detection of an underperforming implantable cardiovascular device using an automated safety surveillance tool. Circ Cardiovasc Qual Outcomes. 3-1-2012;5:189-196. *PMID: 22396584*

132. Landolina, M., Gasparini, M., Lunati, M., Iacopino, S., Boriani, G., Bonanno, C., Vado, A., Proclemer, A., Capucci, A., Zucchiatti, C., Valsecchi, S., Ricci, R. P., Santini, M., and Cardiovascular Centers Participating in the ClinicalService Project. Long-term complications related to biventricular defibrillator implantation: rate of surgical revisions and impact on survival: insights from the Italian Clinical Service Database. Circulation. 6-7-2011;123:2526-2535. *PMID: 21576653*

133. Lee, D. S., Krahn, A. D., Healey, J. S., Birnie, D., Crystal, E., Dorian, P., Simpson, C. S., Khaykin, Y., Cameron, D., Janmohamed, A., Yee, R., Austin, P. C., Chen, Z., Hardy, J., Tu, J. V., and Investigators of the Ontario ICD Database. Evaluation of early complications related to De Novo cardioverter defibrillator implantation insights from the Ontario ICD database. J Am Coll Cardiol. 2-23-2010;55:774-782. *PMID: 20170816*

134. Lyman, S., Sedrakyan, A., Do, H., Razzano, R., and Mushlin, A. I. Infrequent physician use of implantable cardioverter-defibrillators risks patient safety. Heart. 2011;97:1655-1660. *PMID: 21795298*

135. MacFadden, D. R., Crystal, E., Krahn, A. D., Mangat, I., Healey, J. S., Dorian, P., Birnie, D., Simpson, C. S., Khaykin, Y., Pinter, A., Nanthakumar, K., Calzavara, A. J., Austin, P. C., Tu, J. V., and Lee, D. S. Sex differences in implantable cardioverter-defibrillator outcomes: findings from a prospective defibrillator database. Ann Intern Med. 2-7-2012;156:195-203. *PMID: 22312139*

136. Morrison, T. B., Friedman, P. A., Kallinen, L. M., Hodge, D. O., Crusan, D., Kumar, K., Hayes, D. L., Rea, R. F., and Hauser, R. G. Impact of implanted recalled sprint Fidelis lead on patient mortality. J Am Coll Cardiol. 7-12-2011;58:278-283. *PMID: 21737019*

137. Porterfield, J. G., Porterfield, L. M., Kuck, K. H., Corbisiero, R., Greenberg, S. M., Hindricks, G., Wazni, O., Beau, S. L., and Herre, J. M. Clinical performance of the St. Jude Medical Riata defibrillation lead in a large patient population. J Cardiovasc Electrophysiol. 2010;21:551-556. *PMID: 19925609*

138. Remmelts, H. H., Meine, M., Loh, P., Hauer, R., Doevendans, P. A., van Herwerden, L. A., Hopmans, T. E., and Ellerbroek, P. M. Infection after ICD implantation: operating room versus cardiac catheterisation laboratory. Neth Heart J. 2009;17:95-100. *PMID: 19325900*

139. Thijssen, J., Borleffs, C. J., van Rees, J. B., Man, S., de Bie, M. K., Venlet, J., van der Velde, E. T., van, Erven L., and Schalij, M. J. Implantable cardioverter-defibrillator longevity under clinical circumstances: an analysis according to device type, generation, and manufacturer. Heart Rhythm. 2012;9:513-519. *PMID: 22094073*

140. Tsai, F. S., Aronow, W. S., Devabhaktuni, S., Desai, H., Kruger, A., Lai, H. M., Frishman, W. H., Cohen, M., and Sorbera, C. Prevalence of complications during implantation and during 38-month follow-up of 1060 consecutive patients with implantable cardioverter-defibrillators. Am J Ther. 2010;17:e8-10. *PMID: 19262366*

141. van Rees, J. B., van Welsenes, G. H., Borleffs, C. J., Thijssen, J., van der Velde, E. T., van der Wall, E. E., van, Erven L., and Schalij, M. J. Update on small-diameter implantable cardioverter-defibrillator leads performance. Pacing Clin Electrophysiol. 2012;35:652-658. *PMID: 22352338*

142. Varma, N., Michalski, J., Epstein, A. E., and Schweikert, R. Automatic remote monitoring of implantable cardioverter-defibrillator lead and generator performance: the Lumos-T Safely RedUceS RouTine Office Device Follow-Up (TRUST) trial. Circ Arrhythm Electrophysiol. 10-1-2010;3:428-436. *PMID: 20716717*

143. Bode, F., Himmel, F., Reppel, M., Mortensen, K., Schunkert, H., and Wiegand, U. K. Should all dysfunctional high-voltage leads be extracted? Results of a single-centre long-term registry. Europace. 2012;14:1764-1770. *PMID: 22753865*

144. Cheung, J. W., Tobin-Hess, A., Patel, A., Slotwiner, D. J., and Goldner, B. G. Trends in Fidelis lead survival: transition from an exponential to linear pattern of lead failure over time. Circ.Arrhythm.Electrophysiol. 2012;5:906-912. *PMID: 22923271*

145. Freudenberger, R. S., Hellkamp, A. S., Halperin, J. L., Poole, J., Anderson, J., Johnson, G., Mark, D. B., Lee, K. L., and Bardy, G. H. Risk of thromboembolism in heart failure: an analysis from the Sudden Cardiac Death in Heart Failure Trial (SCD-HeFT). Circulation. 5-22-2007;115:2637-2641. *PMID: 17485579*

146. Sengupta, J., Kendig, A. C., Goormastic, M., Hwang, E. S., Ching, E. A., Chung, R., Lindsay, B. D., Tchou, P. J., Wilkoff, B. L., Niebauer, M. J., Martin, D. O., Varma, N., Wazni, O., Saliba, W., Kanj, M., Bhargava, M., Dresing, T., Taigen, T., Ingelmo, C., Bassiouny, M., Cronin, E. M., Wilsmore, B., Rickard, J., and Chung, M. K. Implantable cardioverter-defibrillator FDA safety advisories: Impact on patient mortality and morbidity. Heart Rhythm. 2012;9:1619-1626. *PMID: 22772136*

147. Tzogias, L., Bellavia, D., Sharma, S., Donohue, T. J., and Schoenfeld, M. H. Natural history of the Sprint Fidelis lead: survival analysis from a large single-center study. J.Interv.Card Electrophysiol. 2012;34:37-44. *PMID: 22314669*

148. [Position of the Swiss Nursing Association to the report on "Home nursing from the viewpoint of the social insurances". Formulate the aims positively]. Krankenpfl.Soins.Infirm. 1992;85:74-75. *PMID: 1597965*

149. Parkash, R., Thibault, B., Sterns, L., Sapp, J., Krahn, A., Talajic, M., Luce, M., Yetisir, E., Theoret-Patrick, P., Wells, G., and Tang, A. Sprint Fidelis lead fractures in patients with cardiac resynchronization therapy devices: insight from the Resynchronization/Defibrillation for Ambulatory Heart Failure (RAFT) study. Circulation. 12-18-2012;126:2928-2934. *PMID: 23159551*

150. Martin, D. T., McNitt, S., Nesto, R. W., Rutter, M. K., and Moss, A. J. Cardiac resynchronization therapy reduces the risk of cardiac events in patients with diabetes enrolled in the multicenter automatic defibrillator implantation trial with cardiac resynchronization therapy (MADIT-CRT). Circ Heart Fail. 2011;4:332-338. *PMID: 21350054*

151. van Rees, J. B., Borleffs, C. J., Thijssen, J., de Bie, M. K., van, Erven L., Cannegieter, S. C., Bax, J. J., and Schalij, M. J. Prophylactic implantable cardioverter-defibrillator treatment in the elderly: therapy, adverse events, and survival gain. Europace. 2012;14:66-73. *PMID: 21920909*

152. Desai, H., Aronow, W. S., Ahn, C., Gandhi, K., Hussain, S., Lai, H. M., Sharma, M., Frishman, W. H., Cohen, M., and Sorbera, C. Risk factors for appropriate cardioverter-defibrillator shocks, inappropriate cardioverter-defibrillator shocks, and time to mortality in 549 patients with heart failure. Am J Cardiol. 5-1-2010;105:1336-1338. *PMID: 20403488*

153. Kleemann, T., Hochadel, M., Strauss, M., Skarlos, A., Seidl, K., and Zahn, R. Comparison Between Atrial Fibrillation-Triggered Implantable Cardioverter-Defibrillator (ICD) Shocks and Inappropriate Shocks Caused by Lead Failure: Different Impact on Prognosis in Clinical Practice. J Cardiovasc Electrophysiol. 2012;23:735-740. *PMID: 22313314*

154. Larsen, P. D., De, Silva P., Harding, S. A., Woodcock, E., and Lever, N. A. Use of implantable cardioverter defibrillators in the New Zealand context from 2000 to 2007. N Z Med J. 2-19-2010;123:76-85. *PMID: 20186244*

155. Sandesara, C. M., Sullivan, R. M., Russo, A. M., Li, W., Kendig, A., Day, J. D., Mullin, C., Stolen, K., and Olshansky, B. Older persons with diabetes receive fewer inappropriate ICD shocks: results from the INTRINSIC RV trial. J Cardiovasc Transl Res. 2011;4:27-34. *PMID: 21086086*

156. Saxon, L. A., Hayes, D. L., Gilliam, F. R., Heidenreich, P. A., Day, J., Seth, M., Meyer, T. E., Jones, P. W., and Boehmer, J. P. Long-term outcome after ICD and CRT implantation and influence of remote device follow-up: the ALTITUDE survival study. Circulation. 12-7-2010;122:2359-2367. *PMID: 21098452*

157. Schaer, B., Sticherling, C., Szili-Torok, T., Osswald, S., Jordaens, L., and Theuns, D. A. Impact of left ventricular ejection fraction on occurrence of ventricular events in defibrillator patients with coronary artery disease. Europace. 2011;13:1562-1567. *PMID: 21712284*

158. Sweeney, M. O., Sherfesee, L., DeGroot, P. J., Wathen, M. S., and Wilkoff, B. L. Differences in effects of electrical therapy type for ventricular arrhythmias on mortality in implantable cardioverter-defibrillator patients. Heart Rhythm. 2010;7:353-360. *PMID: 20185109*

159. van Welsenes, G. H., van Rees, J. B., Borleffs, C. J., Cannegieter, S. C., Bax, J. J., van, Erven L., and Schalij, M. J. Long-term follow-up of primary and secondary prevention implantable cardioverter defibrillator patients. Europace. 2011;13:389-394. *PMID: 21208947*

160. Gold, M. R., Ahmad, S., Browne, K., Berg, K. C., Thackeray, L., and Berger, R. D. Prospective comparison of discrimination algorithms to prevent inappropriate ICD therapy: primary results of the Rhythm ID Going Head to Head Trial. Heart Rhythm. 2012;9:370-377. *PMID: 21978966*

161. Sweeney, M. O., Sakaguchi, S., Simons, G., Machado, C., Connett, J. E., Yang, F., and OMNI, Study, I. Response to the Center for Medicare & Medicaid Services coverage with evidence development request for primary prevention implantable cardioverter-defibrillators: Data from the OMNI study. Heart Rhythm. 2012;9:1058-1066. *PMID: 22387371*

162. van Rees, J. B., Borleffs, C. J., de Bie, M. K., Stijnen, T., van, Erven L., Bax, J. J., and Schalij, M. J. Inappropriate implantable cardioverter-defibrillator shocks: incidence, predictors, and impact on mortality. J Am Coll Cardiol. 2-1-2011;57:556-562. *PMID: 21272746*

163. Bigger, J. T., Jr., Whang, W., Rottman, J. N., Kleiger, R. E., Gottlieb, C. D., Namerow, P. B., Steinman, R. C., and Estes, N. A., III. Mechanisms of death in the CABG Patch trial: a randomized trial of implantable cardiac defibrillator prophylaxis in patients at high risk of death after coronary artery bypass graft surgery. Circulation. 3-23-1999;99:1416-1421. *PMID: 10086963*

164. Ghanbari, Hamid, Dalloul, Ghassan, Hasan, Reema, Daccarett, Marcos, Saba, Souheil, David, Shukri, and Machado, Christian. Effectiveness of Implantable Cardioverter-Defibrillators for the Primary Prevention of Sudden Cardiac Death in Women With Advanced Heart Failure: A Meta-analysis of Randomized Controlled Trials. Archives of Internal Medicine. 9-14-2009;169:1500-1506. *PMID: 19752408*

165. Santangeli, P., Pelargonio, G., Dello, Russo A., Casella, M., Bisceglia, C., Bartoletti, S., Santarelli, P., Di, Biase L., and Natale, A. Gender differences in clinical outcome and primary prevention defibrillator benefit in patients with severe left ventricular dysfunction: a systematic review and meta-analysis. Heart Rhythm. 2010;7:876-882. *PMID: 20380893*

166. Buxton, A. E., Lee, K. L., Fisher, J. D., Josephson, M. E., Prystowsky, E. N., and Hafley, G. A randomized study of the prevention of sudden death in patients with coronary artery disease. Multicenter Unsustained Tachycardia Trial Investigators. N.Engl.J.Med. 12-16-1999;341:1882-1890. *PMID: 10601507*

167. Moss, A. J., Hall, W. J., Cannom, D. S., Klein, H., Brown, M. W., Daubert, J. P., Estes, N. A., III, Foster, E., Greenberg, H., Higgins, S. L., Pfeffer, M. A., Solomon, S. D., Wilber, D., Zareba, W., and MADIT-CRT Trial Investigators. Cardiac-resynchronization therapy for the prevention of heart-failure events. New England Journal of Medicine. 10-1-2009;361:1329-1338. *PMID: 19723701*

168. Schuger, C., Daubert, J. P., Brown, M. W., Cannom, D., Estes, N. A., III, Hall, W. J., Kayser, T., Klein, H., Olshansky, B., Power, K. A., Wilber, D., Zareba, W., and Moss, A. J. Multicenter automatic defibrillator implantation trial: reduce inappropriate therapy (MADIT-RIT): background, rationale, and clinical protocol. Ann Noninvasive Electrocardiol. 2012;17:176-185. *PMID: 22816536*

169. Masoudi, F. A., Go, A. S., Magid, D. J., Cassidy-Bushrow, A. E., Doris, J. M., Fiocchi, F., Garcia-Montilla, R., Glenn, K. A., Goldberg, R. J., Gupta, N., Gurwitz, J. H., Hammill, S. C., Hayes, J. J., Jackson, N., Kadish, A., Lauer, M., Miller, A. W., Multerer, D., Peterson, P. N., Reifler, L. M., Reynolds, K., Saczynski, J. S., Schuger, C., Sharma, P. P., Smith, D. H., Suits, M., Sung, S. H., Varosy, P. D., Vidaillet, H. J., and Greenlee, R. T. Longitudinal study of implantable cardioverter-defibrillators: methods and clinical characteristics of patients receiving implantable cardioverter-defibrillators for primary prevention in contemporary practice. Circ.Cardiovasc.Qual.Outcomes. 2012;5:e78-e85. *PMID: 23170006*

170. Nanthakumar, K., Epstein, A. E., Kay, G. N., Plumb, V. J., and Lee, D. S. Prophylactic implantable cardioverter-defibrillator therapy in patients with left ventricular systolic dysfunction: a pooled analysis of 10 primary prevention trials. J.Am.Coll.Cardiol. 12-7-2004;44:2166-2172. *PMID: 15582314*

171. Desai, A. S., Fang, J. C., Maisel, W. H., and Baughman, K. L. Implantable defibrillators for the prevention of mortality in patients with nonischemic cardiomyopathy: a meta-

analysis of randomized controlled trials. JAMA. 12-15-2004;292:2874-2879. *PMID: 15598919*

172. Santangeli, P., Di, Biase L., Dello, Russo A., Casella, M., Bartoletti, S., Santarelli, P., Pelargonio, G., and Natale, A. Meta-analysis: age and effectiveness of prophylactic implantable cardioverter-defibrillators. Ann Intern.Med. 11-2-2010;153:592-599. *PMID: 21041579*

173. Young, J. B., Abraham, W. T., Smith, A. L., Leon, A. R., Lieberman, R., Wilkoff, B., Canby, R. C., Schroeder, J. S., Liem, L. B., Hall, S., and Wheelan, K. Combined cardiac resynchronization and implantable cardioversion defibrillation in advanced chronic heart failure: the MIRACLE ICD Trial. JAMA. 5-28-2003;289:2685-2694. *PMID: 12771115*

174. Beshai, J. F., Grimm, R. A., Nagueh, S. F., Baker, J. H., Beau, S. L., Greenberg, S. M., Pires, L. A., and Tchou, P. J. Cardiac-resynchronization therapy in heart failure with narrow QRS complexes. N.Engl.J.Med. 12-13-2007;357:2461-2471. *PMID: 17986493*

175. Epstein, A. E., Kay, G. N., Plumb, V. J., McElderry, H. T., Doppalapudi, H., Yamada, T., Shafiroff, J., Syed, Z. A., and Shkurovich, S. Implantable cardioverter-defibrillator prescription in the elderly. Heart Rhythm. 2009;6:1136-1143. *PMID: 19539542*

176. Chen, C. Y., Stevenson, L. W., Stewart, G. C., Seeger, J. D., Williams, L., Jalbert, J. J., and Setoguchi, S. Impact of baseline heart failure burden on post-implantable cardioverter-defibrillator mortality among medicare beneficiaries. J Am.Coll.Cardiol. 5-28-2013;61:2142-2150. *PMID: 23541973*

177. Costantini, O., Hohnloser, S. H., Kirk, M. M., Lerman, B. B., Baker, J. H., Sethuraman, B., Dettmer, M. M., and Rosenbaum, D. S. The ABCD (Alternans Before Cardioverter Defibrillator) Trial: strategies using T-wave alternans to improve efficiency of sudden cardiac death prevention. J Am.Coll.Cardiol. 2-10-2009;53:471-479. *PMID: 19195603*

178. FDA approves first subcutaneous heart defibrillator, http://www.fda.gov/NewsEvents/Newsroom/PressAnnouncements/ucm321755.htm, last accessed 1/8/13. 2012

179. Gasparini, M., Proclemer, A., Klersy, C., Kloppe, A., Lunati, M., Ferrer, J. B., Hersi, A., Gulaj, M., Wijfels, M. C., Santi, E., Manotta, L., and Arenal, A. Effect of long-detection interval vs standard-detection interval for implantable cardioverter-defibrillators on antitachycardia pacing and shock delivery: the ADVANCE III randomized clinical trial. JAMA. 5-8-2013;309:1903-1911. *PMID: 23652522*

Appendix A. Search Strategy

Databases:

1) **Ovid MEDLINE** ® 1948 to December Week 1 2012
2) **Ovid MEDLINE** ® **In-Process & Other Non-Indexed Citations** November 30, 2012
3) **EBM Reviews-Cochrane Central Register of Controlled Trials** 4th Quarter 2012

Search Terms:

#	Searches	Brief description of terms	Number of abstracts
1	defibrillators, implantable.sh.	Terms related to device of interest	9,770
2	(defibrillators and implantable).af.		10,520
3	implantable defibrillators.af.		656
4	(implantable and cardioverter and defibrillator).af.		5,507
5	implantable cardioverter defibrillator.af.		4,645
6	cardioverter defibrillators, implantable.af.		1
7	(death, sudden, cardiac and cardiac pacing, artificial).af.	Terms related to outcome of interest	310
8	or/1-7		**11,828**
9	randomized controlled trial.pt.	RCT module	623,823
10	controlled clinical trial.pt		164,766
11	randomized controlled trials/		83,169
12	Random Allocation/		93,931
13	Double-blind Method/		208,115
14	Single-Blind Method/		25,802
15	clinical trial.pt.		745,680
16	Clinical Trials.mp. or exp Clinical Trials/		304,982
17	(clinic$ adj25 trial$).tw.		270,192
18	((singl$ or doubl$ or trebl$ or tripl$) adj (mask$ or blind$)).tw.		238,018
19	Placebos/		50,936
20	placebo$.tw.		253,666
21	random$.tw.		877,789
22	trial$.tw.		687,536
23	(randomized control trial or clinical control trial).sd.		232,482
24	(latin adj square).tw.		3,834
25	Comparative Study.tw. or Comparative Study.pt.		1,718,659
26	exp Evaluation studies/		160,402
27	Follow-Up Studies/		472,156
28	Prospective Studies/		367,536
29	(control$ or prospectiv$ or volunteer$).tw.		2,861,505
30	Cross-Over Studies/		51,220
31	or/9-30		5,503,700
32	8 and 31	Comparative ICD studies	5,457
33	exp cohort studies/ or exp prospective studies/ or exp retrospective studies/ or exp epidemiologic studies/ or exp case-control studies/	Cohort module	1,471,173

34	(cohort or retrospective or prospective or longitudinal or observational or follow-up or followup or registry).af.		1,819,849
35	case-control.af. or (case adj10 control).tw.		175,858
36	ep.fs. *(epidemiology/floating subhead)*		1,046,431
37	or/33-36		2,709,357
38	8 not 31		6,437
39	37 and 38	Cohort ICD studies	*1,309*
40	**32 or 39**	**All ICD studies**	**6,766**

NOTE: The above search strategy was successfully tested against the major RCTs identified in the review by Passman R, Kadish A. Sudden death prevention with implantable devices. *Circulation* 2007:116:561-71; PMID: 17664385.

Appendix B. Excluded Studies

The 223 studies excluded after full-text review are listed in alphabetical order by first author under each main reason for exclusion (bold headings): adverse event paper published before 2002 (n=10), <500 adverse events (n=8), mixed primary and secondary prevention and no adverse effect (n=33), no outcomes of interest (n=28), and not comparison of interest (n=6), not intervention of interest (n=3), outcome numerator or denominator unclear (n=8), protocol (not full article) (n=5), review/editorial (n=4), secondary prevention (n=31), not study design of interest (n=59), wrong population (n=24), and other (n=4). PMIDs are given at the end of each reference, when available.

Adverse Event Paper Published Before 2002 (n=10)

1. Pacifico A, Johnson JW, Stanton MS, et al. Comparison of results in two implantable defibrillators. Jewel 7219D Investigators. Am J Cardiol 1998 Oct 1;82(7):875-80. PMID: 9781970.

2. Hoffmann E, Steinbeck G. Experience with pectoral versus abdominal implantation of a small defibrillator. A multicenter comparison in 778 patients. European Jewel Investigators. Eur Heart J 1998 Jul;19(7):1085-98. PMID: 9717045.

3. Rosenqvist M, Beyer T, Block M, et al. Adverse events with transvenous implantable cardioverter-defibrillators: a prospective multicenter study. European 7219 Jewel ICD investigators. Circulation 1998 Aug 18;98(7):663-70. PMID: 9715859.

4. Smith PN, Vidaillet HJ, Hayes JJ, et al. Infections with nonthoracotomy implantable cardioverter defibrillators: can these be prevented? Endotak Lead Clinical Investigators. Pacing Clin Electrophysiol 1998 Jan;21(1 Pt 1):42-55. PMID: 9474647.

5. Narasimhan C, Dhala A, Axtell K, et al. Comparison of outcome of implantable cardioverter defibrillator implantation in patients with severe versus moderately severe left ventricular dysfunction secondary to atherosclerotic coronary artery disease. Am J Cardiol 1997 Nov 15;80(10):1305-08. PMID: 9388103.

6. Panotopoulos PT, Axtell K, Anderson AJ, et al. Efficacy of the implantable cardioverter-defibrillator in the elderly. J Am Coll Cardiol 1997 Mar 1;29(3):556-60. PMID: 9060893.

7. Gold MR, Peters RW, Johnson JW, et al. Complications associated with pectoral implantation of cardioverter defibrillators. World-Wide Jewel Investigators. Pacing Clin Electrophysiol 1997 Jan;20(1 Pt 2):208-11. PMID: 9121991.

8. Gallik DM, Ben-Zur UM, Gross JN, et al. Lead fracture in cephalic versus subclavian approach with transvenous implantable cardioverter defibrillator systems. Pacing Clin Electrophysiol 1996 Jul;19(7):1089-94. PMID: 8823837.

9. Zipes DP, Roberts D. Results of the international study of the implantable pacemaker cardioverter-defibrillator. A comparison of epicardial and endocardial lead systems. The Pacemaker-Cardioverter-Defibrillator Investigators. Circulation 1995 Jul 1;92(1):59-65. PMID: 7788918.

10. Mosteller RD, Lehmann MH, Thomas AC, et al. Operative mortality with implantation of the automatic cardioverter-defibrillator. Am J Cardiol 1991 Nov 15;68(13):1340-45. PMID: 1951123.

Adverse Events N<500 (n=13)

1. Holst AG, Jensen HK, Eschen O, et al. Low disease prevalence and inappropriate implantable cardioverter defibrillator shock rate in Brugada syndrome: a nationwide study. Europace 2012 Jul;14(7):1025-29. PMID: 22286273.

2. Yu JB, Yang B, Xu DJ, et al. [Impact of metoprolol use in the treatment of patients with electrical-storm after cardioverter defibrillators implantation]. Zhonghua Xin Xue Guan Bing Za Zhi 2011 Aug;39(8):717-20. PMID: 22169417.

3. Forleo GB, Tesauro M, Panattoni G, et al. Impact of continuous intracardiac ST-segment monitoring on mid-term outcomes of ICD-implanted patients with coronary artery disease. Early results of a prospective comparison with conventional ICD outcomes. Heart 2012 Mar;98(5):402-07. PMID: 22115985.

4. Gojkovic O, Aliot EM, Capucci A, et al. Celivarone in patients with an implantable cardioverter-defibrillator: adjunctive therapy for the reduction of ventricular arrhythmia-triggered implantable cardioverter-defibrillator interventions. Heart Rhythm 2012 Feb;9(2):217-24. PMID: 21978965.

5. McLeod CJ, Shen WK, Rea RF, et al. Differential outcome of cardiac resynchronization therapy in ischemic cardiomyopathy and idiopathic dilated cardiomyopathy. Heart Rhythm 2011 Mar;8(3):377-82. PMID: 21070886.

6. Kettering K, Mewis C, Dornberger V, et al. Long-term experience with subcutaneous ICD leads: a comparison among three different types of subcutaneous leads. Pacing Clin Electrophysiol 2004 Oct;27(10):1355-61. PMID: 15511244.

7. Sandstedt B, Kennergren C, Schaumann A, et al. Short- and long-term performance of a tripolar down-sized single lead for implantable cardioverter defibrillator treatment: a randomized prospective European multicenter study. European Endotak DSP Investigator Group. Pacing Clin Electrophysiol 1998 Nov;21(11 Pt 1):2087-94. PMID: 9826861.

8. Mehta D, Nayak HM, Singson M, et al. Late complications in patients with pectoral defibrillator implants with transvenous defibrillator lead systems: high incidence of insulation breakdown. Pacing Clin Electrophysiol 1998 Oct;21(10):1893-900. PMID: 9793085.

9. Lelakowski J, Piekarz J, Rydlewska A, et al. Determinants of patient survival rate after implantation of a cardioverter-defibrillator without resynchronisation capability. Kardiol Pol 2012;70(11):1099-110. PMID: 23180517.

10. Codner P, Nevzorov R, Kusniec J, et al. Implantable cardioverter defibrillator with and without defibrillation threshold testing. Isr Med Assoc J 2012 Jun;14(6):343-46. PMID: 22891393.

11. Aschenbrenner T, Brockmeier J, Bramlage P, et al. Improved survival of patients with coronary artery disease and low ejection fraction with ICD implantation versus conventional therapy in a real world survey. BMC Res Notes 2012;5:382. PMID: 22840219.

12. Lovelock JD, Patel A, Mengistu A, et al. Generator exchange is associated with an increased rate of Sprint Fidelis lead failure. Heart Rhythm 2012 Oct;9(10):1615-18. PMID: 22683747.

13. Clementy N, Pierre B, Lallemand B, et al. Long-term follow-up on high-rate cut-off programming for implantable cardioverter defibrillators in primary prevention patients with left ventricular systolic dysfunction. Europace 2012 Jul;14(7):968-74. PMID: 22389416.

Mixed Primary and Secondary Prevention, No Adverse Effect (n=33)

1. Pedersen SS, Tekle FB, Hoogwegt MT, et al. Shock and patient preimplantation type D personality are associated with poor health status in patients with implantable cardioverter-defibrillator. Circ Cardiovasc Qual Outcomes 2012 May;5(3):373-80. PMID: 22570357.

2. Cho EY, von KR, Marten-Mittag B, et al. Determinants and trajectory of phobic anxiety in patients living with an implantable cardioverter defibrillator. Heart 2012 May;98(10):806-12. PMID: 22543838.

3. Berg SK, Higgins M, Reilly CM, et al. Sleep quality and sleepiness in persons with implantable cardioverter defibrillators: outcome from a clinical randomized longitudinal trial. Pacing Clin Electrophysiol 2012 Apr;35(4):431-43. PMID: 22303998.

4. Shalaby A, Brumberg G, El-Saed A, et al. Mood disorders and outcome in patients receiving cardiac resynchronization therapy. Pacing Clin Electrophysiol 2012 Mar;35(3):294-301. PMID: 22229659.

5. Flemme I, Johansson I, Stromberg A. Living with life-saving technology - coping strategies in implantable cardioverter defibrillators recipients. J Clin Nurs 2012 Feb;21(3-4):311-21. PMID: 21951323.

6. Habibovic M, van den Broek KC, Alings M, et al. Posttraumatic stress 18 months following cardioverter defibrillator implantation: shocks, anxiety, and personality. Health Psychol 2012 Mar;31(2):186-93. PMID: 21806300.

7. Pedersen SS, Hoogwegt MT, Jordaens L, et al. Relation of symptomatic heart failure and psychological status to persistent depression in patients with implantable cardioverter-defibrillator. Am J Cardiol 2011 Jul 1;108(1):69-74. PMID: 21529736.

8. Tzeis S, Kolb C, Baumert J, et al. Effect of depression on mortality in implantable cardioverter defibrillator recipients--findings from the prospective LICAD study. Pacing Clin Electrophysiol 2011 Aug;34(8):991-97. PMID: 21438895.

9. Chair SY, Lee CK, Choi KC, et al. Quality of life outcomes in chinese patients with implantable cardioverter defibrillators. Pacing Clin Electrophysiol 2011 Jul;34(7):858-67. PMID: 21410723.

10. Heatherly SJ, Simmons T, Fitzgerald DM, et al. Psychological effects of implantable cardioverter-defibrillator leads under advisory. Pacing Clin Electrophysiol 2011 Jun;34(6):694-99. PMID: 21410721.

11. von KR, Baumert J, Kolb C, et al. Chronic posttraumatic stress and its predictors in patients living with an implantable cardioverter defibrillator. J Affect Disord 2011 Jun;131(1-3):344-52. PMID: 21195483.

12. Marcus GM, Chan DW, Redberg RF. Recollection of pain due to inappropriate versus appropriate implantable cardioverter-defibrillator shocks. Pacing Clin Electrophysiol 2011 Mar;34(3):348-53. PMID: 21077915.

13. Suzuki T, Shiga T, Kuwahara K, et al. Prevalence and persistence of depression in patients with implantable cardioverter defibrillator: a 2-year longitudinal study. Pacing Clin Electrophysiol 2010 Dec;33(12):1455-61. PMID: 20946285.

14. Keren A, Sears SF, Nery P, et al. Psychological adjustment in ICD patients living with advisory fidelis leads.

J Cardiovasc Electrophysiol 2011 Jan;22(1):57-63. PMID: 20731739.

15. Pedersen SS, van den Broek KC, Erdman RA, et al. Pre-implantation implantable cardioverter defibrillator concerns and Type D personality increase the risk of mortality in patients with an implantable cardioverter defibrillator. Europace 2010 Oct;12(10):1446-52. PMID: 20719779.

16. Dickerson SS, Kennedy M, Wu YW, et al. Factors related to quality-of-life pattern changes in recipients of implantable defibrillators. Heart Lung 2010 Nov;39(6):466-76. PMID: 20561848.

17. Pedersen SS, Theuns DA, Jordaens L, et al. Course of anxiety and device-related concerns in implantable cardioverter defibrillator patients the first year post implantation. Europace 2010 Aug;12(8):1119-26. PMID: 20507853.

18. Kapa S, Rotondi-Trevisan D, Mariano Z, et al. Psychopathology in patients with ICDs over time: results of a prospective study. Pacing Clin Electrophysiol 2010 Feb;33(2):198-208. PMID: 19930108.

19. Pedersen SS, den Broek KC, Theuns DA, et al. Risk of chronic anxiety in implantable defibrillator patients: a multi-center study. Int J Cardiol 2011 Mar 17;147(3):420-23. PMID: 19896732.

20. Kim J, Pressler SJ, Welch JL, et al. Validity and reliability of the chronic heart failure questionnaire mastery subscale in patients with defibrillators. West J Nurs Res 2009 Dec;31(8):1057-75. PMID: 19783791.

21. Pinter A, Mangat I, Korley V, et al. Assessment of resynchronization therapy on functional status and quality of life in patients requiring an implantable defibrillator. Pacing Clin Electrophysiol 2009 Dec;32(12):1509-19. PMID: 19765233.

22. Fisher JD, Koulogiannis KP, Lewallen L, et al. The psychological impact of implantable cardioverter-defibrillator recalls and the durable positive effects of counseling. Pacing Clin Electrophysiol 2009 Aug;32(8):1012-16. PMID: 19659621.

23. van den Broek KC, Nyklicek I, Van d, V, et al. Risk of ventricular arrhythmia after implantable defibrillator treatment in anxious type D patients. J Am Coll Cardiol 2009 Aug 4;54(6):531-37. PMID: 19643315.

24. Pandya K, Patel MB, Natla J, et al. Predictors of hemodynamic compromise with propofol during defibrillator implantation: a single center experience. J Interv Card Electrophysiol 2009 Aug;25(2):145-51. PMID: 19263205.

25. Bilge AK, Ozben B, Demircan S, et al. Depression and anxiety status of patients with implantable cardioverter defibrillator and precipitating factors. Pacing Clin Electrophysiol 2006 Jun;29(6):619-26. PMID: 16784428.

26. Wathen MS, DeGroot PJ, Sweeney MO, et al. Prospective randomized multicenter trial of empirical antitachycardia pacing versus shocks for spontaneous rapid ventricular tachycardia in patients with implantable cardioverter-defibrillators: Pacing Fast Ventricular Tachycardia Reduces Shock Therapies (PainFREE Rx II) trial results. Circulation 2004 Oct 26;110(17):2591-96. PMID: 15492306.

27. Pedersen SS, van Domburg RT, Theuns DA, et al. Type D personality is associated with increased anxiety and depressive symptoms in patients with an implantable cardioverter defibrillator and their partners. Psychosom Med 2004 Sep;66(5):714-19. PMID: 15385696.

28. Shukla HH, Flaker GC, Jayam V, et al. High defibrillation thresholds in transvenous biphasic implantable defibrillators: clinical predictors and prognostic implications. Pacing Clin Electrophysiol 2003 Jan;26(1 Pt 1):44-48. PMID: 12685138.

29. Godemann F, Ahrens B, Behrens S, et al. Classic conditioning and dysfunctional cognitions in patients with panic disorder and agoraphobia treated with an implantable cardioverter/defibrillator. Psychosom Med 2001 Mar;63(2):231-38. PMID: 11292270.

30. Duru F, Buchi S, Klaghofer R, et al. How different from pacemaker patients are recipients of implantable cardioverter-defibrillators with respect to psychosocial adaptation, affective disorders, and quality of life? Heart 2001 Apr;85(4):375-79. PMID: 11250956.

31. Herbst JH, Goodman M, Feldstein S, et al. Health-related quality-of-life assessment of patients with life-threatening ventricular arrhythmias. Pacing Clin Electrophysiol 1999 Jun;22(6 Pt 1):915-26. PMID: 10392390.

32. Pacifico A, Hohnloser SH, Williams JH, et al. Prevention of implantable-defibrillator shocks by treatment with sotalol. d,l-Sotalol Implantable Cardioverter-Defibrillator Study Group. N Engl J Med 1999 Jun 17;340(24):1855-62. PMID: 10369848.

33. Dunbar SB, Jenkins LS, Hawthorne M, et al. Mood disturbance in patients with recurrent ventricular dysrhythmia before insertion of implantable cardioverter defibrillator. Heart Lung 1996 Jul;25(4):253-61. PMID: 8836741.

No Outcomes of Interest (n=43)

1. Barsheshet A, Moss AJ, Huang DT, et al. Applicability of a risk score for prediction of the long-term (8-year) benefit of the implantable cardioverter-defibrillator. J Am Coll Cardiol 2012 Jun 5;59(23):2075-79. PMID: 22651863.

2. George J, Barsheshet A, Moss AJ, et al. Effectiveness of cardiac resynchronization therapy in diabetic patients with ischemic and nonischemic cardiomyopathy. Ann Noninvasive Electrocardiol 2012 Jan;17(1):14-21. PMID: 22276624.

3. Versteeg H, Starrenburg A, Denollet J, et al. Monitoring device acceptance in implantable cardioverter defibrillator patients using the Florida Patient Acceptance Survey. Pacing Clin Electrophysiol 2012 Mar;35(3):283-93. PMID: 22229519.

4. Zecchin M, Merlo M, Pivetta A, et al. How can optimization of medical treatment avoid unnecessary implantable cardioverter-defibrillator implantations in patients with idiopathic dilated cardiomyopathy presenting with "SCD-HeFT criteria?". Am J Cardiol 2012 Mar 1;109(5):729-35. PMID: 22176998.

5. Sullivan RM, Russo AM, Berg KC, et al. Arrhythmia rate distribution and tachyarrhythmia therapy in an ICD population: results from the INTRINSIC RV trial. Heart Rhythm 2012 Mar;9(3):351-58. PMID: 22016074.

6. Hoogwegt MT, Kupper N, Theuns DA, et al. Beta-blocker therapy is not associated with symptoms of depression and anxiety in patients receiving an implantable cardioverter-defibrillator. Europace 2012 Jan;14(1):74-80. PMID: 21920910.

7. Sohail MR, Henrikson CA, Braid-Forbes MJ, et al. Mortality and cost associated with cardiovascular implantable electronic device infections. Arch Intern Med 2011 Nov 14;171(20):1821-28. PMID: 21911623.

8. Goldenberg I, Moss AJ, Hall WJ, et al. Predictors of response to cardiac resynchronization therapy in the Multicenter Automatic Defibrillator Implantation Trial with Cardiac Resynchronization Therapy (MADIT-

CRT). Circulation 2011 Oct 4;124(14):1527-36. PMID: 21900084.

9. Buber J, Klein H, Moss AJ, et al. Clinical course and outcome of patients enrolled in US and non-US centres in MADIT-CRT. Eur Heart J 2011 Nov;32(21):2697-704. PMID: 21642283.

10. Barsheshet A, Goldenberg I, Moss AJ, et al. Effect of elapsed time from coronary revascularization to implantation of a cardioverter defibrillator on long-term survival in the MADIT-II trial. J Cardiovasc Electrophysiol 2011 Nov;22(11):1237-42. PMID: 21615813.

11. Pouleur AC, Knappe D, Shah AM, et al. Relationship between improvement in left ventricular dyssynchrony and contractile function and clinical outcome with cardiac resynchronization therapy: the MADIT-CRT trial. Eur Heart J 2011 Jul;32(14):1720-29. PMID: 21609974.

12. Knappe D, Pouleur AC, Shah AM, et al. Dyssynchrony, contractile function, and response to cardiac resynchronization therapy. Circ Heart Fail 2011 Jul;4(4):433-40. PMID: 21602574.

13. Perrotta L, Pieragnoli P, Ricciardi G, et al. Multicenter experience with implantable defibrillators subject to recall. Pacing Clin Electrophysiol 2011 Aug;34(8):998-1002. PMID: 21438897.

14. Rordorf R, Canevese F, Vicentini A, et al. Delayed ICD lead cardiac perforation: comparison of small versus standard-diameter leads implanted in a single center. Pacing Clin Electrophysiol 2011 Apr;34(4):475-83. PMID: 21208240.

15. Linde C, Mealing S, Hawkins N, et al. Cost-effectiveness of cardiac resynchronization therapy in patients with asymptomatic to mild heart failure: insights from the European cohort of the REVERSE (Resynchronization Reverses remodeling in Systolic Left Ventricular Dysfunction). Eur Heart J

2011 Jul;32(13):1631-39. PMID: 21112898.

16. Barsheshet A, Goldenberg I, Moss AJ, et al. Response to preventive cardiac resynchronization therapy in patients with ischaemic and nonischaemic cardiomyopathy in MADIT-CRT. Eur Heart J 2011 Jul;32(13):1622-30. PMID: 21075774.

17. Barsheshet A, Moss AJ, Eldar M, et al. Time-dependent benefit of preventive cardiac resynchronization therapy after myocardial infarction. Eur Heart J 2011 Jul;32(13):1614-21. PMID: 21075773.

18. Sauer WH, Lowery CM, Bargas RL, et al. Utility of postoperative testing of implantable cardioverter-defibrillators. Pacing Clin Electrophysiol 2011 Feb;34(2):186-92. PMID: 21039640.

19. Goldenberg I, Moss AJ, McNitt S, et al. Relation between renal function and response to cardiac resynchronization therapy in Multicenter Automatic Defibrillator Implantation Trial--Cardiac Resynchronization Therapy (MADIT-CRT). Heart Rhythm 2010 Dec;7(12):1777-82. PMID: 20833266.

20. Mohamad T, Jacob S, Kommuri NV, et al. Low referral pattern for implantable defibrillator therapy in a tertiary hospital: referral physician survey and Monte Carlo simulation. Am J Ther 2011 Sep;18(5):350-54. PMID: 20335787.

21. Sumner AD, Boehmer JP, Saxon LA, et al. Statin use is associated with improved survival in patients with advanced heart failure receiving resynchronization therapy. Congest Heart Fail 2009 Jul;15(4):159-64. PMID: 19627288.

22. Saxon LA, Olshansky B, Volosin K, et al. Influence of left ventricular lead location on outcomes in the COMPANION study. J Cardiovasc Electrophysiol 2009 Jul;20(7):764-68. PMID: 19298563.

23. Belardinelli R, Capestro F, Misiani A, et al. Moderate exercise training improves functional capacity, quality of life, and endothelium-dependent vasodilation in chronic heart failure patients with implantable cardioverter defibrillators and cardiac resynchronization therapy. Eur J Cardiovasc Prev Rehabil 2006 Oct;13(5):818-25. PMID: 17001224.

24. Steinbeck G, Andresen D, Senges J, et al. Immediate Risk-Stratification Improves Survival (IRIS): study protocol. Europace 2004 Sep;6(5):392-99. PMID: 15294263.

25. Lampert R, Joska T, Burg MM, et al. Emotional and physical precipitants of ventricular arrhythmia. Circulation 2002 Oct 1;106(14):1800-05. PMID: 12356633.

26. Schulte B, Sperzel J, Carlsson J, et al. Dual-coil vs single-coil active pectoral implantable defibrillator lead systems: defibrillation energy requirements and probability of defibrillation success at multiples of the defibrillation energy requirements. Europace 2001 Jul;3(3):177-80. PMID: 11467457.

27. Whang W, Bigger JT, Jr. Diabetes and outcomes of coronary artery bypass graft surgery in patients with severe left ventricular dysfunction: results from The CABG Patch Trial database. The CABG Patch Trial Investigators and Coordinators. J Am Coll Cardiol 2000 Oct;36(4):1166-72. PMID: 11028466.

28. Bigger JT, Jr., Whang W, Rottman JN, et al. Mechanisms of death in the CABG Patch trial: a randomized trial of implantable cardiac defibrillator prophylaxis in patients at high risk of death after coronary artery bypass graft surgery. Circulation 1999 Mar 23;99(11):1416-21. PMID: 10086963.

29. Masoudi FA, Go AS, Magid DJ, et al. Longitudinal study of implantable cardioverter-defibrillators: methods and clinical characteristics of patients receiving implantable cardioverter-defibrillators for primary prevention in contemporary practice. Circ Cardiovasc Qual Outcomes 2012 Nov;5(6):e78-e85. PMID: 23170006.

30. Veazie PJ, Noyes K, Li Q, et al. Cardiac resynchronization and quality of life in patients with minimally symptomatic heart failure. J Am Coll Cardiol 2012 Nov 6;60(19):1940-44. PMID: 23062542.

31. Bilchick KC, Stukenborg GJ, Kamath S, et al. Prediction of mortality in clinical practice for medicare patients undergoing defibrillator implantation for primary prevention of sudden cardiac death. J Am Coll Cardiol 2012 Oct 23;60(17):1647-55. PMID: 23021331.

32. Flo GL, Glenny RW, Kudenchuk PJ, et al. Development and safety of an exercise testing protocol for patients with an implanted cardioverter defibrillator for primary or secondary indication. Cardiopulm Phys Ther J 2012 Sep;23(3):16-22. PMID: 22993498.

33. Hsu JC, Solomon SD, Bourgoun M, et al. Predictors of super-response to cardiac resynchronization therapy and associated improvement in clinical outcome: the MADIT-CRT (multicenter automatic defibrillator implantation trial with cardiac resynchronization therapy) study. J Am Coll Cardiol 2012 Jun 19;59(25):2366-73. PMID: 22698490.

34. Barsheshet A, Moss AJ, Huang DT, et al. Applicability of a risk score for prediction of the long-term (8-year) benefit of the implantable cardioverter-defibrillator. J Am Coll Cardiol 2012 Jun 5;59(23):2075-79. PMID: 22651863.

35. Leenhardt A, Defaye P, Mouton E, et al. First inappropriate implantable cardioverter defibrillator therapy is often due to inaccurate device programming: analysis of the French OPERA registry. Europace 2012 Oct;14(10):1465-74. PMID: 22547767.

36. Martins RP, Blangy H, Muresan L, et al. Safety and efficacy of programming a

high number of antitachycardia pacing attempts for fast ventricular tachycardia: a prospective study. Europace 2012 Oct;14(10):1457-64. PMID: 22547765.

37. Brenyo A, Goldenberg I, Moss AJ, et al. Baseline functional capacity and the benefit of cardiac resynchronization therapy in patients with mildly symptomatic heart failure enrolled in MADIT-CRT. Heart Rhythm 2012 Sep;9(9):1454-59. PMID: 22521920.

38. Ji SY, Gundewar S, Palma EC. Subclavian venoplasty may reduce implant times and implant failures in the era of increasing device upgrades. Pacing Clin Electrophysiol 2012 Apr;35(4):444-48. PMID: 22229641.

39. Sullivan RM, Russo AM, Berg KC, et al. Arrhythmia rate distribution and tachyarrhythmia therapy in an ICD population: results from the INTRINSIC RV trial. Heart Rhythm 2012 Mar;9(3):351-58. PMID: 22016074.

40. Kramer DB, Friedman PA, Kallinen LM, et al. Development and validation of a risk score to predict early mortality in recipients of implantable cardioverter-defibrillators. Heart Rhythm 2012 Jan;9(1):42-46. PMID: 21893137.

41. Fischer A, Ousdigian KT, Johnson JW, et al. The impact of atrial fibrillation with rapid ventricular rates and device programming on shocks in 106,513 ICD and CRT-D patients. Heart Rhythm 2012 Jan;9(1):24-31. PMID: 21835150.

42. Atary JZ, Borleffs CJ, van der Bom JG, et al. Right ventricular stimulation threshold at ICD implant predicts device therapy in primary prevention patients with ischaemic heart disease. Europace 2010 Nov;12(11):1581-88. PMID: 20639206.

43. Borleffs CJ, van Rees JB, van Welsenes GH, et al. Prognostic importance of atrial fibrillation in implantable cardioverter-defibrillator patients. J Am Coll Cardiol 2010 Mar 2;55(9):879-85. PMID: 20185038.

Not Comparison of Interest (n=6)

1. Gilliam FR, Hayes DL, Boehmer JP, et al. Real world evaluation of dual-zone ICD and CRT-D programming compared to single-zone programming: the ALTITUDE REDUCES study. J Cardiovasc Electrophysiol 2011 Sep;22(9):1023-29. PMID: 21627705.
   Comparison: programming

2. Hauser RG, Maisel WH, Friedman PA, et al. Longevity of Sprint Fidelis implantable cardioverter-defibrillator leads and risk factors for failure: implications for patient management. Circulation 2011 Feb 1;123(4):358-63. PMID: 21242478.
   Comparison: lead 1 vs. lead 2

3. Russo AM, Hafley GE, Lee KL, et al. Racial differences in outcome in the Multicenter UnSustained Tachycardia Trial (MUSTT): a comparison of whites versus blacks. Circulation 2003 Jul 8;108(1):67-72. PMID: 12821551.
   Outcome not based on ICD vs. no ICD

4. Wilkoff BL, Cook JR, Epstein AE, et al. Dual-chamber pacing or ventricular backup pacing in patients with an implantable defibrillator: the Dual Chamber and VVI Implantable Defibrillator (DAVID) Trial. JAMA 2002 Dec 25;288(24):3115-23. PMID: 12495391.
   Comparison: programming

5. Kohn CS, Petrucci RJ, Baessler C, et al. The effect of psychological intervention on patients' long-term adjustment to the ICD: a prospective study. Pacing Clin Electrophysiol 2000 Apr;23(4 Pt 1):450-56. PMID: 10793433.
   Comparison: Psych. therapy vs. control

6. Giorgberidze I, Saksena S, Krol RB, et al. Risk stratification and clinical outcome of minimally symptomatic and

asymptomatic patients with nonsustained ventricular tachycardia and coronary disease: a prospective

single-center study. Am J Cardiol 1997 Sep 11;80(5B):3F-9F. PMID: 9291444. *Comparison: ICD or drug 1 vs. drug 2*

Not Intervention of Interest (n=3)

1. Rodriguez Y, Garisto JD, Carrillo RG. Laser lead extraction in the octogenarian patient. Circ Arrhythm Electrophysiol 2011 Oct;4(5):719-23. PMID: 22007037.
Lead extraction

2. Mela T, McGovern BA, Garan H, et al. Long-term infection rates associated with the pectoral versus abdominal approach to cardioverter- defibrillator implants. Am J Cardiol 2001 Oct

1;88(7):750-53. PMID: 11589841. *Abdominal implants*

3. Buxton AE, Lee KL, Fisher JD, et al. A randomized study of the prevention of sudden death in patients with coronary artery disease. Multicenter Unsustained Tachycardia Trial Investigators. N Engl J Med 1999 Dec 16;341(25):1882-90. PMID: 10601507.
Not an ICD trial

Outcome Numerator or Denominator Unclear (n=8)

1. Duggirala HJ, Herz ND, Canos DA, et al. Disproportionality analysis for signal detection of implantable cardioverter-defibrillator-related adverse events in the Food and Drug Administration Medical Device Reporting System. Pharmacoepidemiol Drug Saf 2012 Jan;21(1):87-93. PMID: 22095760.

2. Smith T, van Dessel PF, Theuns DA, et al. Health care utilisation after defibrillator implantation for primary prevention according to the guidelines in 2 Dutch academic medical centres. Neth Heart J 2011 Oct;19(10):405-11. PMID: 21773744.

3. Rodriguez Y, Baltodano P, Tower A, et al. Management of symptomatic inadvertently placed endocardial leads in the left ventricle. Pacing Clin Electrophysiol 2011 Oct;34(10):1192-200. PMID: 21671951.

4. van G, I, Phan HM, Wilkoff BL, et al. Prognostic significance of atrial arrhythmias in a primary prevention ICD population. Pacing Clin Electrophysiol 2011 Sep;34(9):1070-79. PMID: 21605131.

5. Smit J, Korup E, Schonheyder HC. Infections associated with permanent pacemakers and implanted cardioverter-defibrillator devices. A 10-year regional study in Denmark. Scand J Infect Dis 2010 Sep;42(9):658-64. PMID: 20465488.

6. Santini M, Lunati M, Defaye P, et al. Prospective multicenter randomized trial of fast ventricular tachycardia termination by prolonged versus conventional anti-tachyarrhythmia burst pacing in implantable cardioverter-defibrillator patients-Atp DeliVery for pAiNless ICD thErapy (ADVANCE-D) Trial results. J Interv Card Electrophysiol 2010 Mar;27(2):127-35. PMID: 20087760.

7. Wilkoff BL, Williamson BD, Stern RS, et al. Strategic programming of detection and therapy parameters in implantable cardioverter-defibrillators reduces shocks in primary prevention patients: results from the PREPARE (Primary Prevention Parameters Evaluation) study. J Am Coll Cardiol 2008 Aug 12;52(7):541-50. PMID: 18687248.

8. Wilkoff BL, Ousdigian KT, Sterns LD, et al. A comparison of empiric to physician-

tailored programming of implantable cardioverter-defibrillators: results from the prospective randomized multicenter

EMPIRIC trial. J Am Coll Cardiol 2006 Jul 18;48(2):330-39. PMID: 16843184.

Protocol (n=6)

1. Pedersen SS, Lambiase P, Boersma LV, et al. Evaluation oF FactORs ImpacTing CLinical Outcome and Cost EffectiveneSS of the S-ICD: design and rationale of the EFFORTLESS S-ICD Registry. Pacing Clin Electrophysiol 2012 May;35(5):574-79. PMID: 22360677.

2. Pedersen SS, Spek V, Theuns DA, et al. Rationale and design of WEBCARE: a randomized, controlled, web-based behavioral intervention trial in cardioverter-defibrillator patients to reduce anxiety and device concerns and enhance quality of life. Trials 2009;10:120. PMID: 20030843.

3. Moss AJ, Brown MW, Cannom DS, et al. Multicenter automatic defibrillator implantation trial-cardiac resynchronization therapy (MADIT-CRT): design and clinical protocol. Ann

Noninvasive Electrocardiol 2005 Oct;10(4 Suppl):34-43. PMID: 16274414.

4. Moss AJ et al. Multicenter automatic defibrillator implantation trial II (MADIT II): design and clinical protocol. Ann Noninvasive Electrocardiol. 2012

5. Kadish A, Quigg R, Schaechter A, et al. Defibrillators in nonischemic cardiomyopathy treatment evaluation. Pacing Clin Electrophysiol 2000 Mar;23(3):338-43. PMID: 10750134.

6. Schuger C, Daubert JP, Brown MW, et al. Multicenter automatic defibrillator implantation trial: reduce inappropriate therapy (MADIT-RIT): background, rationale, and clinical protocol. Ann Noninvasive Electrocardiol 2012 Jul;17(3):176-85. PMID: 22816536

Review/Editorial (n=4)

1. Atwater BD, Daubert JP. Implantable cardioverter defibrillators: risks accompany the life-saving benefits. Heart 2012 May;98(10):764-72. PMID: 22422588.

2. Gasparini M, Nisam S. Implantable cardioverter defibrillator harm? Europace 2012 Aug;14(8):1087-93. PMID: 22389417.

3. Kelly D, Mariathas M, Gough R, et al. Is a new high-voltage lead necessary? 6.6-

French ICD lead failure: a UK tertiary center experience. Pacing Clin Electrophysiol 2012 Jan;35(1):1-2. PMID: 22077138.

4. Salukhe TV, Francis DP, Sutton R. Comparison of medical therapy, pacing and defibrillation in heart failure (COMPANION) trial terminated early; combined biventricular pacemaker-defibrillators reduce all-cause mortality and hospitalization. Int J Cardiol 2003 Feb;87(2-3):119-20. PMID: 12559527.

Secondary Prevention (n=31)

1. Ye S, Grunnert M, Thune JJ, et al. Circumstances and outcomes of sudden

unexpected death in patients with high-risk myocardial infarction: implications for prevention. Circulation 2011 Jun 14;123(23):2674-80. PMID: 21606398.

2. Redhead AP, Turkington D, Rao S, et al. Psychopathology in postinfarction patients implanted with cardioverter-defibrillators for secondary prevention. A cross-sectional, case-controlled study. J Psychosom Res 2010 Dec;69(6):555-63. PMID: 21109043.

3. Hallas CN, Burke JL, White DG, et al. A prospective 1-year study of changes in neuropsychological functioning after implantable cardioverter-defibrillator surgery. Circ Arrhythm Electrophysiol 2010 Apr;3(2):170-77. PMID: 20197542.

4. MacFadden DR, Tu JV, Chong A, et al. Evaluating sex differences in population-based utilization of implantable cardioverter-defibrillators: role of cardiac conditions and noncardiac comorbidities. Heart Rhythm 2009 Sep;6(9):1289-96. PMID: 19695966.

5. Bagherzadeh A, Emkanjoo Z, Haghjoo M, et al. Complications and mortality of single versus dual chamber implantable cardioverter defibrillators. Indian Pacing Electrophysiol J 2006;6(2):75-83. PMID: 16943899.

6. Kron J. Clinical significance of device-related complications in clinical trials and implications for future trials: insights from the Antiarrhytmics Versus Implantable Defibrillators (AVID) trial. Card Electrophysiol Rev 2003 Dec;7(4):473-78. PMID: 15071278.

7. Kamphuis HC, de L, Jr., Derksen R, et al. Implantable cardioverter defibrillator recipients: quality of life in recipients with and without ICD shock delivery: a prospective study. Europace 2003 Oct;5(4):381-89. PMID: 14753636.

8. Young JB, Abraham WT, Smith AL, et al. Combined cardiac resynchronization and implantable cardioversion defibrillation in advanced chronic heart failure: the MIRACLE ICD Trial. JAMA 2003 May 28;289(20):2685-94. PMID: 12771115.

9. Fries R, Konig J, Schafers HJ, et al. Triggering effect of physical and mental stress on spontaneous ventricular tachyarrhythmias in patients with implantable cardioverter-defibrillators. Clin Cardiol 2002 Oct;25(10):474-78. PMID: 12375806.

10. Hsu J, Uratsu C, Truman A, et al. Life after a ventricular arrhythmia. Am Heart J 2002 Sep;144(3):404-12. PMID: 12228776.

11. Takahashi T, Bhandari AK, Watanuki M, et al. High incidence of device-related and lead-related complications in the dual-chamber implantable cardioverter defibrillator compared with the single-chamber version. Circ J 2002 Aug;66(8):746-50. PMID: 12197599.

12. Pires LA, Sethuraman B, Guduguntla VD, et al. Outcome of women versus men with ventricular tachyarrhythmias treated with the implantable cardioverter defibrillator. J Cardiovasc Electrophysiol 2002 Jun;13(6):563-68. PMID: 12108497.

13. Cook JR, Rizo-Patron C, Curtis AB, et al. Effect of surgical revascularization in patients with coronary artery disease and ventricular tachycardia or fibrillation in the Antiarrhythmics Versus Implantable Defibrillators (AVID) Registry. Am Heart J 2002 May;143(5):821-26. PMID: 12040343.

14. Della BP. [Canadian Implantable Defibrillator Study (CIDS): a randomized trial of the implantable cardioverter defibrillator against amiodarone]. Ital Heart J Suppl 2000 Aug;1(8):1070-71. PMID: 10993020.

15. Connolly SJ, Gent M, Roberts RS, et al. Canadian implantable defibrillator study (CIDS) : a randomized trial of the implantable cardioverter defibrillator against amiodarone. Circulation 2000 Mar 21;101(11):1297-302. PMID: 10725290.

16. Dunbar SB, Kimble LP, Jenkins LS, et al. Association of mood disturbance and

arrhythmia events in patients after cardioverter defibrillator implantation. Depress Anxiety 1999;9(4):163-68. PMID: 10431681.

17. Trappe HJ, Achtelik M, Pfitzner P, et al. Single-chamber versus dual-chamber implantable cardioverter defibrillators: indications and clinical results. Am J Cardiol 1999 Mar 11;83(5B):8D-16D. PMID: 10089834.

18. Heller SS, Ormont MA, Lidagoster L, et al. Psychosocial outcome after ICD implantation: a current perspective. Pacing Clin Electrophysiol 1998 Jun;21(6):1207-15. PMID: 9633062.

19. Bourke JP, Turkington D, Thomas G, et al. Florid psychopathology in patients receiving shocks from implanted cardioverter-defibrillators. Heart 1997 Dec;78(6):581-83. PMID: 9470875.

20. Schuster PM, Phillips S, Dillon DL, et al. The psychosocial and physiological experiences of patients with an implantable cardioverter defibrillator. Rehabil Nurs 1998 Jan;23(1):30-37. PMID: 9460456.

21. Domanski MJ, Saksena S, Wyse G, et al. Clinical and socioeconomic profile of patients with malignant ventricular arrhythmias in 1993 to 1995. AVID investigators. Antiarrhythmics Versus Implantable Defibrillator. Am J Cardiol 1997 Aug 1;80(3):299-301. PMID: 9264422.

22. Hegel MT, Griegel LE, Black C, et al. Anxiety and depression in patients receiving implanted cardioverter-defibrillators: a longitudinal investigation. Int J Psychiatry Med 1997;27(1):57-69. PMID: 9565714.

23. Haffajee C, Martin D, Bhandari A, et al. A multicenter, randomized trial comparing an active can implantable defibrillator with a passive can system. Jewel Active Can Investigators. Pacing Clin Electrophysiol 1997 Jan;20(1 Pt 2):215-19. PMID: 9121993.

24. Ector H, Jordaens L, Vanhaecke J. Survival analysis and clinical medicine. An observational comparison of the implantable cardioverter defibrillator, amiodarone treatment, and heart transplantation. Eur Heart J 1996 Sep;17(9):1444-47. PMID: 8880032.

25. Fleurant E, Lacroix D, Klug D, et al. [Automatic implantable defibrillator and antiarrhythmic surgery in ischemic cardiopathies. Apropos of 53 cases]. Arch Mal Coeur Vaiss 1995 Nov;88(11):1627-34. PMID: 8745998.

26. Arteaga WJ, Windle JR. The quality of life of patients with life-threatening arrhythmias. Arch Intern Med 1995 Oct 23;155(19):2086-91. PMID: 7575068.

27. Clinical outcome of patients with malignant ventricular tachyarrhythmias and a multiprogrammable implantable cardioverter-defibrillator implanted with or without thoracotomy: an international multicenter study. PCD Investigator Group. J Am Coll Cardiol 1994 Jun;23(7):1521-30. PMID: 8195508.

28. Trappe HJ, Klein H, Wenzlaff P, et al. Role of interventional therapy in patients with coronary heart disease and life-threatening ventricular tachyarrhythmias. Eur Heart J 1993 Sep;14 Suppl E:120-27. PMID: 8223748.

29. Gross JN, Sackstein RD, Song SL, et al. The antitachycardia pacing ICD: impact on patient selection and outcome. Pacing Clin Electrophysiol 1993 Jan;16(1 Pt 2):165-69. PMID: 7681565.

30. Pinski SL, Mick MJ, Arnold AZ, et al. Retrospective analysis of patients undergoing one- or two-stage strategies for myocardial revascularization and implantable cardioverter defibrillator implantation. Pacing Clin Electrophysiol 1991 Jul;14(7):1138-47. PMID: 1715551.

31. Thomas AC, Moser SA, Smutka ML, et al. Implantable defibrillation: eight years clinical experience. Pacing Clin Electrophysiol 1988 Nov;11(11 Pt 2):2053-58. PMID: 2463587.

Not Study Design of Interest (n=66)

1. Hickman RL, Jr., Pinto MD, Lee E, et al. Exploratory and confirmatory factor analysis of the decision regret scale in recipients of internal cardioverter defibrillators. J Nurs Meas 2012;20(1):21-34. PMID: 22679707. *Reason for Exclusion: cross-sectional*

2. van Rees JB, Borleffs CJ, van Welsenes GH, et al. Clinical prediction model for death prior to appropriate therapy in primary prevention implantable cardioverter defibrillator patients with ischaemic heart disease: the FADES risk score. Heart 2012 Jun;98(11):872-77. PMID: 22581736. *Reason for Exclusion: Cohort study, no adverse events or N<500*

3. Carroll SL, Markle-Reid M, Ciliska D, et al. Age and mental health predict early device-specific quality of life in patients receiving prophylactic implantable defibrillators. Can J Cardiol 2012 Jul;28(4):502-07. PMID: 22425267. *Reason for Exclusion: Cohort study, no adverse events or N<500*

4. Bruggenjurgen B, Israel CW, Klesius AA, et al. Health services research in heart failure patients treated with a remote monitoring device in Germany-a retrospective database analysis in evaluating resource use. J Med Econ 2012;15(4):737-45. PMID: 22409232. *Reason for Exclusion: Cohort study, no adverse events or N<500*

5. Ziegler PD, Koehler JL, Verma A. Continuous versus intermittent monitoring of ventricular rate in patients with permanent atrial fibrillation. Pacing Clin Electrophysiol 2012 May;35(5):598-604. PMID: 22394432. *Reason for Exclusion: Cohort study, no adverse events or N<500*

6. James CA, Tichnell C, Murray B, et al. General and disease-specific psychosocial adjustment in patients with arrhythmogenic right ventricular dysplasia/cardiomyopathy with implantable cardioverter defibrillators: a large cohort study. Circ Cardiovasc Genet 2012 Feb 1;5(1):18-24. PMID: 22238189. *Reason for Exclusion: Cohort study, no adverse events or N<500*

7. Epstein AJ, Polsky D, Yang F, et al. Geographic variation in implantable cardioverter-defibrillator use and heart failure survival. Med Care 2012 Jan;50(1):10-17. PMID: 22167063. *Reason for Exclusion: Cohort study, no adverse events or N<500*

8. Scott PA, Whittaker A, Zeb M, et al. Rates of upgrade of ICD recipients to CRT in clinical practice and the potential impact of the more liberal use of CRT at initial implant. Pacing Clin Electrophysiol 2012 Jan;35(1):73-80. PMID: 22054072. *Reason for Exclusion: Cohort study, no adverse events or N<500*

9. Cesarino CB, Beccaria LM, Aroni MM, et al. Quality of life of patients with implantable cardioverser-defibrillator: the usage of SF-36 questionnaire. Rev Bras Cir Cardiovasc 2011 Apr;26(2):238-43. PMID: 21894414. *Reason for Exclusion: Cohort study, no adverse events or N<500*

10. Kramer DB, Friedman PA, Kallinen LM, et al. Development and validation of a risk score to predict early mortality in recipients of implantable cardioverter-defibrillators. Heart Rhythm 2012 Jan;9(1):42-46. PMID: 21893137. *Reason for Exclusion: Cohort study, no adverse events or N<500*

11. Sack S, Wende CM, Nagele H, et al. Potential value of automated daily screening of cardiac resynchronization therapy defibrillator diagnostics for prediction of major cardiovascular events: results from Home-CARE (Home Monitoring in Cardiac Resynchronization Therapy) study. Eur J Heart Fail 2011 Sep;13(9):1019-27. PMID: 21852311. *Reason for Exclusion: Cohort study, no adverse events or N<500*

12. Fischer A, Ousdigian KT, Johnson JW, et al. The impact of atrial fibrillation with rapid ventricular rates and device programming on shocks in 106,513 ICD and CRT-D patients. Heart Rhythm 2012 Jan;9(1):24-31. PMID: 21835150. *Reason for Exclusion: Cohort study, no adverse events or N<500*

13. Lazarus A, Biondi N, Thebaut JF, et al. Implantable cardioverter-defibrillators in France: practices and regional variability. Europace 2011 Nov;13(11):1568-73. PMID: 21784742. *Reason for Exclusion: cross-sectional*

14. Tavenaux M, Ginzburg DM, Boukacem A, et al. [Changes in depression, anxiety, and vital exhaustion in patients after ICD implantation. Comparison of clinical subgroups]. Herzschrittmacherther Elektrophysiol 2011 Sep;22(3):174-79. PMID: 21773789. *Reason for Exclusion: Cohort study, no adverse events or N<500*

15. Pedersen SS, Versteeg H, Nielsen JC, et al. Patient-reported outcomes in Danish implantable cardioverter defibrillator patients with a Sprint Fidelis lead advisory notification. Europace 2011 Sep;13(9):1292-98. PMID: 21616945. *Reason for Exclusion: cross-sectional*

16. Flemme I, Hallberg U, Johansson I, et al. Uncertainty is a major concern for patients with implantable cardioverter defibrillators. Heart Lung 2011 Sep;40(5):420-28. PMID: 21459446. *Reason for Exclusion: Cohort study, no adverse events or N<500*

17. Probst V, Plassard-Kerdoncuf D, Mansourati J, et al. The psychological impact of implantable cardioverter defibrillator implantation on Brugada syndrome patients. Europace 2011 Jul;13(7):1034-39. PMID: 21427091. *Reason for Exclusion: Cohort study, no adverse events or N<500*

18. Mellert F, Schneider C, Esmailzadeh B, et al. Implantation of left ventricular epicardial leads in cardiosurgical patients with impaired cardiac function-- a worthwhile procedure in concomitant surgical interventions? Thorac Cardiovasc Surg 2012 Feb;60(1):64-69. PMID: 21425053. *Reason for Exclusion: Cohort study, no adverse events or N<500*

19. Alla VM, Anand K, Hundal M, et al. Impact of moderate to severe renal impairment on mortality and appropriate shocks in patients with implantable cardioverter defibrillators. Cardiol Res Pract 2010;2010:150285. PMID: 21197424. *Reason for Exclusion: Cohort study, no adverse events or N<500*

20. Cross NJ, McCrae CS, Smith KM, et al. Comparison of actigraphic and subjective measures of sleep in implantable cardioverter defibrillator and coronary artery disease patients. Clin Cardiol 2010 Dec;33(12):753-59. PMID: 21184559. *Reason for Exclusion: Cohort study, no adverse events or N<500*

21. Arnous S, Murphy NF, Pyne-Daly P, et al. Clinical and psychological impact of prophylactic implantable cardioverter-defibrillators in a community heart failure population. Ir J Med Sci 2011 Jun;180(2):369-74. PMID: 21153928. *Reason for Exclusion: Cohort study, no adverse events or N<500*

22. Leistner DM, Schmitt J, Palm S, et al. Intracoronary administration of bone marrow-derived mononuclear cells and arrhythmic events in patients with chronic heart failure. Eur Heart J 2011 Feb;32(4):485-91. PMID: 21138937. *Reason for Exclusion: Cohort study, no adverse events or N<500*

23. Bilchick KC, Kamath S, DiMarco JP, et al. Bundle-branch block morphology and other predictors of outcome after cardiac resynchronization therapy in Medicare patients. Circulation 2010 Nov 16;122(20):2022-30. PMID: 21041691. *Reason for Exclusion: Cohort study, no adverse events or N<500*

24. Hager CS, Jain S, Blackwell J, et al. Effect of renal function on survival after implantable cardioverter defibrillator placement. Am J Cardiol 2010 Nov 1;106(9):1297-300. PMID: 21029827. *Reason for Exclusion: Cohort study, no adverse events or N<500*

25. Versteeg H, Baumert J, Kolb C, et al. Somatosensory amplification mediates sex differences in psychological distress among cardioverter-defibrillator patients. Health Psychol 2010 Sep;29(5):477-83. PMID: 20836602. *Reason for Exclusion: cross-sectional*

26. Chen TB, Cheng KA, Gao P, et al. Primary prevention of sudden cardiac death by implantable cardioverter-defibrillator therapy in Chinese patients with heart failure: a single-center experience. Chin Med J (Engl) 2010 Apr 5;123(7):848-51. PMID: 20497676. *Reason for Exclusion: Cohort study, no adverse events or N<500*

27. Marijon E, Trinquart L, Otmani A, et al. Predictors for short-term progressive heart failure death in New York Heart Association II patients implanted with a cardioverter defibrillator--the EVADEF study. Am Heart J 2010 Apr;159(4):659-64. PMID: 20362726. *Reason for Exclusion: Cohort study, no adverse events or N<500*

28. Salukhe TV, Briceno NI, Ferenczi EA, et al. Is there benefit in implanting defibrillators in patients with severe heart failure? Heart 2010 Apr;96(8):599-603. PMID: 20357388. *Reason for Exclusion: Cohort study, no adverse events or N<500*

29. Desai H, Aronow WS, Ahn C, et al. Incidence of appropriate cardioverter-defibrillator shocks and mortality in patients with heart failure treated with combined cardiac resynchronization plus implantable cardioverter-defibrillator therapy versus implantable cardioverter-defibrillator therapy. J Cardiovasc Pharmacol Ther 2010 Mar;15(1):37-40. PMID: 19966176. *Reason for Exclusion: Cohort study, no adverse events or N<500*

30. Borleffs CJ, van Welsenes GH, van Bommel RJ, et al. Mortality risk score in primary prevention implantable cardioverter defibrillator recipients with non-ischaemic or ischaemic heart disease. Eur Heart J 2010 Mar;31(6):712-18. PMID: 19933693. *Reason for Exclusion: Cohort study, no adverse events or N<500*

31. Kim JS, Pressler SJ, Welch JL, et al. Physical function of patients with implantable cardioverter-defibrillators. J Cardiovasc Nurs 2009 Sep;24(5):398-409. PMID: 19707100. *Reason for Exclusion: Cohort study, no adverse events or N<500*

32. Otmani A, Trinquart L, Marijon E, et al. Rates and predictors of appropriate implantable cardioverter-defibrillator therapy delivery: results from the EVADEF cohort study. Am Heart J 2009 Aug;158(2):230-37. PMID: 19619699. *Reason for Exclusion: Cohort study, no adverse events or N<500*

33. Srivatsa UN, Hoppe BL, Narayan S, et al. Ventricular arrhythmia discriminator programming and the impact on the incidence of inappropriate therapy in patients with implantable cardiac defibrillators. Indian Pacing Electrophysiol J 2007;7(2):77-84. PMID:

17538699. *Reason for Exclusion: Cohort study, no adverse events or N<500*

34. Baumert J, Schmitt C, Ladwig KH. Psychophysiologic and affective parameters associated with pain intensity of cardiac cardioverter defibrillator shock discharges. Psychosom Med 2006 Jul;68(4):591-97. PMID: 16868269. *Reason for Exclusion: cross-sectional*

35. Klein T, Schonecke O, Wollny H, et al. [Clinical significance of stress reactivity for frequency of electric shock discharges in patients with implanted cardioverter-defibrillators]. Dtsch Med Wochenschr 2004 Oct 22;129(43):2291-94. PMID: 15483767. *Reason for Exclusion: Cohort study, no adverse events or N<500*

36. Godemann F, Butter C, Lampe F, et al. Panic disorders and agoraphobia: side effects of treatment with an implantable cardioverter/defibrillator. Clin Cardiol 2004 Jun;27(6):321-26. PMID: 15237689. *Reason for Exclusion: Cohort study, no adverse events or N<500*

37. Ricci R, Quesada A, Pignalberi C, et al. Dual defibrillator improves quality of life and decreases hospitalizations in patients with drug refractory atrial fibrillation. J Interv Card Electrophysiol 2004 Feb;10(1):85-92. PMID: 14739755. *Reason for Exclusion: Cohort study, no adverse events or N<500*

38. Hamilton GA, Carroll DL. The effects of age on quality of life in implantable cardioverter defibrillator recipients. J Clin Nurs 2004 Feb;13(2):194-200. PMID: 14723671. *Reason for Exclusion: Cohort study, no adverse events or N<500*

39. Carroll DL, Hamilton GA, Kenney BJ. Changes in health status, psychological distress, and quality of life in implantable cardioverter defibrillator recipients between 6 months and 1 year after

implantation. Eur J Cardiovasc Nurs 2002 Oct;1(3):213-19. PMID: 14622676. *Reason for Exclusion: Cohort study, no adverse events or N<500*

40. Bolse K, Flemme I, Ivarsson A, et al. Life situation related to the ICD implantation; self-reported uncertainty and satisfaction in Swedish and US samples. Eur J Cardiovasc Nurs 2002 Dec;1(4):243-51. PMID: 14622654. *Reason for Exclusion: Cohort study, no adverse events or N<500*

41. Pelletier D, Gallagher R, Mitten-Lewis S, et al. Australian implantable cardiac defibrillator recipients: quality-of-life issues. Int J Nurs Pract 2002 Apr;8(2):68-74. PMID: 11993579. *Reason for Exclusion: Cohort study, no adverse events or N<500*

42. Flemme I, Bolse K, Ivarsson A, et al. Life situation of patients with an implantable cardioverter defibrillator: a descriptive longitudinal study. J Clin Nurs 2001 Jul;10(4):563-72. PMID: 11822504. *Reason for Exclusion: Cohort study, no adverse events or N<500*

43. Wathen MS, Sweeney MO, DeGroot PJ, et al. Shock reduction using antitachycardia pacing for spontaneous rapid ventricular tachycardia in patients with coronary artery disease. Circulation 2001 Aug 14;104(7):796-801. PMID: 11502705. *Reason for Exclusion: Cohort study, no adverse events or N<500*

44. Ahmad M, Bloomstein L, Roelke M, et al. Patients' attitudes toward implanted defibrillator shocks. Pacing Clin Electrophysiol 2000 Jun;23(6):934-38. PMID: 10879375. *Reason for Exclusion: Cohort study, no adverse events or N<500*

45. Pelletier D, Mitten-Lewis S, Gallagher RD, et al. Implantable defibrillator recipients' responses to device implantation and design. Biomed Instrum Technol 1999 May;33(3):224-29. PMID: 10360211. *Reason for*

Exclusion: Cohort study, no adverse events or N<500

46. Pauli P, Wiedemann G, Dengler W, et al. Anxiety in patients with an automatic implantable cardioverter defibrillator: what differentiates them from panic patients? Psychosom Med 1999 Jan;61(1):69-76. PMID: 10024069. *Reason for Exclusion: Cohort study, no adverse events or N<500*

47. Grubman EM, Pavri BB, Shipman T, et al. Cardiac death and stored electrograms in patients with third-generation implantable cardioverter-defibrillators. J Am Coll Cardiol 1998 Oct;32(4):1056-62. PMID: 9768732. *Reason for Exclusion: Cohort study, no adverse events or N<500*

48. Crow SJ, Collins J, Justic M, et al. Psychopathology following cardioverter defibrillator implantation. Psychosomatics 1998 Jul;39(4):305-10. PMID: 9691699. *Reason for Exclusion: Cohort study, no adverse events or N<500*

49. Craney JM, Mandle CL, Munro BH, et al. Implantable cardioverter defibrillators: physical and psychosocial outcomes. Am J Crit Care 1997 Nov;6(6):445-51. PMID: 9354222. *Reason for Exclusion: Cohort study, no adverse events or N<500*

50. Jessurun ER, Hutten BA, van Hemel NM, et al. [Good experiences with an implantable automatic defibrillator with transvenous electrodes for patients with life-threatening arrhythmias]. Ned Tijdschr Geneeskd 1997 Jul 26;141(30):1475-80. PMID: 9542881. *Reason for Exclusion: Cohort study, no adverse events or N<500*

51. Herrmann C, von zur MF, Schaumann A, et al. Standardized assessment of psychological well-being and quality-of-life in patients with implanted defibrillators. Pacing Clin Electrophysiol 1997 Jan;20(1 Pt 1):95-103. PMID: 9121977. *Reason for Exclusion: Cohort study, no adverse events or N<500*

52. Li H, Axtell K, Biehl M, et al. Sudden death in patients with implantable cardioverter-defibrillators. Am Heart J 1996 Nov;132(5):986-88. PMID: 8892772. *Reason for Exclusion: Cohort study, no adverse events or N<500*

53. Jung W, Luderitz B. Quality of life and driving in recipients of the implantable cardioverter-defibrillator. Am J Cardiol 1996 Sep 12;78(5A):51-56. PMID: 8820836. *Reason for Exclusion: Cohort study, no adverse events or N<500*

54. Daoud EG, Strickberger SA, Man KC, et al. Comparison of early and late complications in patients undergoing coronary artery bypass graft surgery with and without concomitant placement of an implantable cardioverter defibrillator. Am Heart J 1995 Oct;130(4):780-85. PMID: 7572586. *Reason for Exclusion: Cohort study, no adverse events or N<500*

55. Vitale MB, Funk M. Quality of life in younger persons with an implantable cardioverter defibrillator. Dimens Crit Care Nurs 1995 Mar;14(2):100-11. PMID: 7889798. *Reason for Exclusion: Cohort study, no adverse events or N<500*

56. Bainger EM, Fernsler JI. Perceived quality of life before and after implantation of an internal cardioverter defibrillator. Am J Crit Care 1995 Jan;4(1):36-43. PMID: 7894553. *Reason for Exclusion: Cohort study, no adverse events or N<500*

57. Luderitz B, Jung W, Deister A, et al. [The quality of life after the implantation of a cardioverter/defibrillator in malignant arrhythmias]. Dtsch Med Wochenschr 1993 Mar 5;118(9):285-89. PMID: 8444109. *Reason for Exclusion: Cohort study, no adverse events or N<500*

58. Nisam S, Mower MM, Thomas A, et al. Patient survival comparison in three generations of automatic implantable cardioverter defibrillators: review of 12 years, 25,000 patients. Pacing Clin

Electrophysiol 1993 Jan;16(1 Pt 2):174-78. PMID: 7681567. *Reason for Exclusion: Cohort study, no adverse events or N<500*

59. Pycha C, Calabrese JR, Gulledge AD, et al. Patient and spouse acceptance and adaptation to implantable cardioverter defibrillators. Cleve Clin J Med 1990 Jul;57(5):441-44. PMID: 2372924. *Reason for Exclusion: Cohort study, no adverse events or N<500*

60. Boriani G, Botto G, Lunati M, et al. Influence of time between last myocardial infarction and prophylactic implantable defibrillator implant on device detections and therapies. "Routine Practice" data from the SEARCH MI registry. BMC Cardiovasc Disord 2012;12:72. PMID: 22966862. *Reason for Exclusion: Cohort study, no adverse events or N<500*

61. Kreuz J, Horlbeck F, Schrickel J, et al. Kidney dysfunction and deterioration of ejection fraction pose independent risk factors for mortality in implantable cardioverter-defibrillator recipients for primary prevention. Clin Cardiol 2012 Sep;35(9):575-79. PMID: 22707222. *Reason for Exclusion: Cohort study, no adverse events or N<500*

62. Parkash R, Sapp JL, Basta M, et al. Use of primary prevention implantable cardioverter-defibrillators in a population-based cohort is associated with a significant survival benefit. Circ Arrhythm Electrophysiol 2012 Aug 1;5(4):706-13. PMID: 22685111.

Reason for Exclusion: historic (not concurrent) control group

63. van Rees JB, Borleffs CJ, van Welsenes GH, et al. Clinical prediction model for death prior to appropriate therapy in primary prevention implantable cardioverter defibrillator patients with ischaemic heart disease: the FADES risk score. Heart 2012 Jun;98(11):872-77. PMID: 22581736. *Reason for Exclusion: Cohort study, no adverse events or N<500*

64. Thijssen J, van Rees JB, Venlet J, et al. The mode of death in implantable cardioverter-defibrillator and cardiac resynchronization therapy with defibrillator patients: results from routine clinical practice. Heart Rhythm 2012 Oct;9(10):1605-12. PMID: 22522066. *Reason for Exclusion: Cohort study, no adverse events or N<500*

65. Carroll SL, Markle-Reid M, Ciliska D, et al. Age and mental health predict early device-specific quality of life in patients receiving prophylactic implantable defibrillators. Can J Cardiol 2012 Jul;28(4):502-07. PMID: 22425267. *Reason for Exclusion: Cohort study, no adverse events or N<500*

66. Biasucci LM, Bellocci F, Landolina M, et al. Risk stratification of ischaemic patients with implantable cardioverter defibrillators by C-reactive protein and a multi-markers strategy: results of the CAMI-GUIDE study. Eur Heart J 2012 Jun;33(11):1344-50. PMID: 22285581. *Reason for Exclusion: Cohort study, no adverse events or N<500*

Wrong Population (n=37)

1. Viola GM, Awan LL, Ostrosky-Zeichner L, et al. Infections of cardiac implantable electronic devices: a retrospective multicenter observational study. Medicine (Baltimore) 2012 May;91(3):123-30. PMID: 22543626.

2. Athan E, Chu VH, Tattevin P, et al. Clinical characteristics and outcome of infective endocarditis involving implantable cardiac devices. JAMA 2012 Apr 25;307(16):1727-35. PMID: 22535857.

3. Deharo JC, Quatre A, Mancini J, et al. Long-term outcomes following infection of cardiac implantable electronic devices: a prospective matched cohort study. Heart 2012 May;98(9):724-31. PMID: 22523057.

4. Powell BD, Asirvatham SJ, Perschbacher DL, et al. Noise, artifact, and oversensing related inappropriate ICD shock evaluation: ALTITUDE noise study. Pacing Clin Electrophysiol 2012 Jul;35(7):863-69. PMID: 22519674.

5. Viganego F, O'Donoghue S, Eldadah Z, et al. Effect of early diagnosis and treatment with percutaneous lead extraction on survival in patients with cardiac device infections. Am J Cardiol 2012 May 15;109(10):1466-71. PMID: 22356796.

6. Greenspon AJ, Prutkin JM, Sohail MR, et al. Timing of the most recent device procedure influences the clinical outcome of lead-associated endocarditis results of the MEDIC (Multicenter Electrophysiologic Device Infection Cohort). J Am Coll Cardiol 2012 Feb 14;59(7):681-87. PMID: 22322085.

7. Jacob S, Panaich SS, Zalawadiya SK, et al. Phantom shocks unmasked: clinical data and proposed mechanism of memory reactivation of past traumatic shocks in patients with implantable cardioverter defibrillators. J Interv Card Electrophysiol 2012 Aug;34(2):205-13. PMID: 22183617.

8. Bogale N, Priori S, Cleland JG, et al. The European CRT Survey: 1 year (9-15 months) follow-up results. Eur J Heart Fail 2012 Jan;14(1):61-73. PMID: 22179034.

9. Bogale N, Witte K, Priori S, et al. The European Cardiac Resynchronization Therapy Survey: comparison of outcomes between de novo cardiac resynchronization therapy implantations and upgrades. Eur J Heart Fail 2011 Sep;13(9):974-83. PMID: 21771823.

10. Le KY, Sohail MR, Friedman PA, et al. Impact of timing of device removal on mortality in patients with cardiovascular implantable electronic device infections. Heart Rhythm 2011 Nov;8(11):1678-85. PMID: 21699855.

11. Tompkins C, McLean R, Cheng A, et al. End-stage renal disease predicts complications in pacemaker and ICD implants. J Cardiovasc Electrophysiol 2011 Oct;22(10):1099-104. PMID: 21489029.

12. Powell BD, Cha YM, Asirvatham SJ, et al. Implantable cardioverter defibrillator electrogram adjudication for device registries: methodology and observations from ALTITUDE. Pacing Clin Electrophysiol 2011 Aug;34(8):1003-12. PMID: 21453341.

13. Sohail MR, Hussain S, Le KY, et al. Risk factors associated with early- versus late-onset implantable cardioverter-defibrillator infections. J Interv Card Electrophysiol 2011 Aug;31(2):171-83. PMID: 21365264.

14. Krahn AD, Lee DS, Birnie D, et al. Predictors of short-term complications after implantable cardioverter-defibrillator replacement: results from the Ontario ICD Database. Circ Arrhythm Electrophysiol 2011 Apr;4(2):136-42. PMID: 21325209.

15. Cengiz M, Okutucu S, Ascioglu S, et al. Permanent pacemaker and implantable cardioverter defibrillator infections: seven years of diagnostic and therapeutic experience of a single center. Clin Cardiol 2010 Jul;33(7):406-11. PMID: 20641117.

16. Tompkins C, Cheng A, Dalal D, et al. Dual antiplatelet therapy and heparin "bridging" significantly increase the risk of bleeding complications after pacemaker or implantable cardioverter-defibrillator device implantation. J Am Coll Cardiol 2010 May 25;55(21):2376-82. PMID: 20488310.

17. Nery PB, Fernandes R, Nair GM, et al. Device-related infection among patients with pacemakers and implantable defibrillators: incidence, risk factors, and consequences. J Cardiovasc Electrophysiol 2010 Jul;21(7):786-90. PMID: 20102431.

18. de Oliveira JC, Martinelli M, Nishioka SA, et al. Efficacy of antibiotic prophylaxis before the implantation of pacemakers and cardioverter-defibrillators: results of a large, prospective, randomized, double-blinded, placebo-controlled trial. Circ Arrhythm Electrophysiol 2009 Feb;2(1):29-34. PMID: 19808441.

19. Curtis LH, Al-Khatib SM, Shea AM, et al. Sex differences in the use of implantable cardioverter-defibrillators for primary and secondary prevention of sudden cardiac death. JAMA 2007 Oct 3;298(13):1517-24. PMID: 17911496.

20. Gunderson BD, Patel AS, Bounds CA, et al. An algorithm to predict implantable cardioverter-defibrillator lead failure. J Am Coll Cardiol 2004 Nov 2;44(9):1898-902. PMID: 15519026.

21. Cabell CH, Heidenreich PA, Chu VH, et al. Increasing rates of cardiac device infections among Medicare beneficiaries: 1990-1999. Am Heart J 2004 Apr;147(4):582-86. PMID: 15077071.

22. Giudici MC, Paul DL, Bontu P, et al. Pacemaker and implantable cardioverter defibrillator implantation without reversal of warfarin therapy. Pacing Clin Electrophysiol 2004 Mar;27(3):358-60. PMID: 15009863.

23. Newman DM, Dorian P, Paquette M, et al. Effect of an implantable cardioverter defibrillator with atrial detection and shock therapies on patient-perceived, health-related quality of life. Am Heart J 2003 May;145(5):841-46. PMID: 12766741.

24. Gronefeld GC, Mauss O, Li YG, et al. Association between atrial fibrillation and appropriate implantable cardioverter defibrillator therapy: results from a prospective study. J Cardiovasc Electrophysiol 2000 Nov;11(11):1208-14. PMID: 11083241.

25. Hua W, Niu H, Fan X, et al. Preventive effectiveness of implantable cardioverter defibrillator in reducing sudden cardiac death in the Chinese population: a multicenter trial of ICD therapy versus non-ICD therapy. J Cardiovasc Electrophysiol 2012 Nov;23 Suppl 1:S5-S9. PMID: 23140347.

26. Dougherty CM, Thompson EA, Kudenchuk PJ. Development and testing of an intervention to improve outcomes for partners following receipt of an implantable cardioverter defibrillator in the patient. ANS Adv Nurs Sci 2012 Oct;35(4):359-77. PMID: 23107992.

27. Chen S, Yin Y, Krucoff MW. Effect of cardiac resynchronization therapy and implantable cardioverter defibrillator on quality of life in patients with heart failure: a meta-analysis. Europace 2012 Nov;14(11):1602-07. PMID: 23104857.

28. Rho RW, Patton KK, Poole JE, et al. Important differences in mode of death between men and women with heart failure who would qualify for a primary prevention implantable cardioverter-defibrillator. Circulation 2012 Nov 13;126(20):2402-07. PMID: 23072904.

29. Healey JS, Hohnloser SH, Exner DV, et al. Cardiac resynchronization therapy in patients with permanent atrial fibrillation: results from the Resynchronization for Ambulatory Heart Failure Trial (RAFT). Circ Heart Fail 2012 Sep 1;5(5):566-70. PMID: 22896584.

30. Ipek EG, Guray U, Demirkan B, et al. Infections of implantable cardiac rhythm devices: predisposing factors and outcome. Acta Cardiol 2012 Jun;67(3):303-10. PMID: 22870738.

31. Brignole M, Occhetta E, Bongiorni MG, et al. Clinical evaluation of defibrillation testing in an unselected population of 2,120 consecutive patients undergoing first implantable cardioverter-defibrillator implant. J Am Coll Cardiol 2012 Sep 11;60(11):981-87. PMID: 22858384.

32. Roig IL, Darouiche RO, Musher DM, et al. Device-related infective endocarditis,

with special consideration of implanted intravascular and cardiac devices in a predominantly male population. Scand J Infect Dis 2012 Oct;44(10):753-60. PMID: 22681242.

33. Hoogwegt MT, Kupper N, Theuns DA, et al. Undertreatment of anxiety and depression in patients with an implantable cardioverter-defibrillator: impact on health status. Health Psychol 2012 Nov;31(6):745-53. PMID: 22545981.

34. Powell BD, Asirvatham SJ, Perschbacher DL, et al. Noise, artifact, and oversensing related inappropriate ICD shock evaluation: ALTITUDE noise study. Pacing Clin Electrophysiol 2012 Jul;35(7):863-69. PMID: 22519674.

35. Boriani G, Santini M, Lunati M, et al. Improving thromboprophylaxis using

atrial fibrillation diagnostic capabilities in implantable cardioverter-defibrillators: the multicentre Italian ANGELS of AF Project. Circ Cardiovasc Qual Outcomes 2012 Mar 1;5(2):182-88. PMID: 22373906.

36. Koopman HM, Vrijmoet-Wiersma CM, Langius JN, et al. Psychological functioning and disease-related quality of life in pediatric patients with an implantable cardioverter defibrillator. Pediatr Cardiol 2012 Apr;33(4):569-75. PMID: 22314365.

37. Marshall P, Ketchell A, Maclean J. Comparison of male and female psychological outcomes related to implantable cardioverter defibrillators (COMFORTID). Eur J Cardiovasc Nurs 2012 Sep;11(3):313-21. PMID: 21802370.

Other (n=4)

1. Sayfo S, Vakil KP, Alqaqa'a A, et al. A retrospective analysis of proceduralist-directed, nurse-administered propofol sedation for implantable cardioverter-defibrillator procedures. Heart Rhythm 2012 Mar;9(3):342-46. PMID: 22001710. *Reason for Exclusion: inpatient adverse effect, not NCDR ICD database*

2. Swindle JP, Rich MW, McCann P, et al. Implantable cardiac device procedures in older patients: use and in-hospital outcomes. Arch Intern Med 2010 Apr 12;170(7):631-37. PMID: 20386008. *Reason for Exclusion: Inpatient adverse effect, not NCDR ICD database*

3. Bhavnani SP, Kluger J, Coleman CI, et al. The prognostic impact of shocks for clinical and induced arrhythmias on morbidity and mortality among patients with implantable cardioverter-defibrillators. Heart Rhythm 2010 Jun;7(6):755-60. PMID: 20211275. *Reason for Exclusion: No data about population*

4. Zaman S, Sivagangabalan G, Narayan A, et al. Outcomes of early risk stratification and targeted implantable cardioverter-defibrillator implantation after ST-elevation myocardial infarction treated with primary percutaneous coronary intervention. Circulation 2009 Jul 21;120(3):194-200. PMID: 19581496. *Reason for Exclusion: intervention arms not comparable*

Appendix C. Supplemental Tables

Appendix Table 1. Baseline data

Study Author, Year PMID	Intervention (Control)	Baseline characteristics Intervention (Control) Age, Y (mean or median)	%Male	%LVEF	%NYHA class	%DM	QRS interval
ICD vs. no ICD							
AMIOVIRT Strickberger, 2003 12767651	ICD (Amiodarone)	58 (60)	67 (74)	22 (23)	Class I: 18 (13); Class II:64 (63); Class III: 16 (24)	31 (36)	nd
CABG-Patch Bigger, 1997 9371853	ICD (No ICD)	64 (63)	87 (82)	27 (27)	Class II or III: 71 (74)	36 (40)	QRS complex >100 msec: 71 (74)
CAT Bansch, 2002 11914254	ICD (Control)	52 (52)	86 (74)	24 (25)	Class II: 67 (64); Class III: 33 (36)	NR	"Abnormal": 27 (45)
Chan, 2009 20031808	ICD (No ICD)	66 (66)	80 (75)	26 (28)	nd	35 (37)	%QRS interval >120 msec: 32 (21)
COMPANION Bristow, 2004 15152059	ICD + CRT (No ICD)	66 (68)	67 (69)	22 (22)	Class III: 86 (82)	41 (45)	160 (158)
DEFINITE Kadish, 2004 15152060	ICD (No ICD)	58 (58)	73 (70)	21 (22)	Class I: 25 (18); Class II: 54 (61); Class III: 21 (21)	23 (23)	115 (116)
Hohnloser, 2004 15590950 DINAMIT	ICD (No ICD)	62 (62)	76 (77)	28 (28)	Class I: 14 (12); Class II:31 (59); Class III: 26 (29)	31 (29)	107 (105)
Fonarow, 2000 10760339	ICD (Control)	49 (48)	68 (58)	21 (21)	Class III: 48 (49); Class IV: 52 (51)	NR	nd
IRIS Steinbeck, 2009 19812399	ICD (No ICD)	63 (62)	78 (76)	NR	At hospital discharge post-MI, the NYHA Class could be assessed in 885 of the surviving patients and was judged to be Class I in 247 patients (28%), Class II in 531 (60%), and Class III in 106 (12%); the Class changed to IV in 1 patient (0.1%).	37 (30)	nd
MADIT Moss, 1996 8960472	ICD (No ICD)	62 (64)	97 (91)	27 (25)	Class II or III: 63 (67)	7 (5)	nd
MADIT II Moss, 2002 11907286	ICD (No ICD)	64 (65)	84 (85)	23 (23)	Class I: 35 (39); Class II:35 (34); Class III: 25 (23); Class IV: 5 (4)	33 (38)	%QRS interval ≥120 msec: 50 (51)

TA on ICD for Primary Prevention
Appendix C

Study Author, Year PMID	Intervention (Control)	Baseline characteristics Intervention (Control)					
		Age, y (mean or median)	%Male	%LVEF	%NYHA class	%DM	QRS interval
Mezu, 2011 21640321	ICD (No ICD)	82 (86)	77 (67)	24 (27)	Class III or IV: 44 (72)	34 (63)	nd
OPTIMIZE-HF and GWTG-H Hernandez, 2010 20009044	ICD (No ICD)	74 (75)	74 (58)	23 (25)	nd	37 (44)	nd
SCD-HeFT Bardy, 2005 15659722	ICD (No ICD/placebo)	60 (60)	77 (76)	Median: 24 (25)	nd	31 (29)	nd
ICD vs. CRT-D							
Diab, 2011 21700757	ICD (CRT-D)	65 (67)	90 (88)	27 (25)	Class III: 89 (88) Mean: 3.2 (3.1)	NR	142 (134)
MADIT-CRT Moss, 2009 19723701	ICD (CRT-D)	64 (65)	76 (75)	24 (24)	Class I (all ischemic): 16 (14); Class II (ischemic): 39 (41); Class II (nonischemic): 45 (45)	31 (30)	%QRS duration ≥150 msec: 65 (64)
MENDMI Chung, 2010 20852059	ICD (CRT-D)	55 (58)	68 (81)	29 (28)	Class I: 16 (17); Class II: 34 (29); Class III: 34 (38); Unknown: 16 (17)	11 (5)	91 (86)
RAFT Tang, 2010 21073365	ICD (CRT-D)	66 (66)	81 (85)	23 (23)	Class II: 81 (79); Class III: 19(21)	35 (33)	Intrinsic: 158 (157); Paced: 210 (207)

AMIOVERT=Amiodarone versus Implantable Cardioverter-Defibrillator Randomized Trial, CABG-Patch=Coronary Artery Bypass Graft Patch, CAT=Cardiomyopathy Trial, COMPANION=Comparison of Medical Therapy, Pacing and Defibrillation in Heart Failure, CRT-D=cardiac resynchronization therapy defibrillator, DEFINITE=Defibrillators in Nonischemic Cardiomyopathy Treatment Evaluation, DINAMIT=Defibrillator in Acute Myocardial Infarction Trial, DM=diabetes, GWTG-HF= Get With the Guidelines-Heart Failure, ICD=implantable cardiac defibrillator, IRIS=Immediate Risk Stratification Improves Survival, LVEF=left ventricular ejection fraction, MADIT=Multicenter Automatic Defibrillator Implantation Trial, MADIT-CRT=Multicenter Automatic Defibrillator Implantation Trial with Cardiac Resynchronization Therapy, MENCMI=Prevention of Myocardial Enlargement and Dilation Post Myocardial Infarction Study, MI= myocardial infarction, msec, millisecond, nd=not documented, NYHA=New York Heart Association, OPTIMIZE-HF=Organized Program to Initiate Lifesaving Treatment in Hospitalized Patients with Heart Failure, SCD-HeFT= Sudden Cardiac Death in Heart Failure Trial, VT=ventricular tachycardia

Appendix Table 2. Concomitant medications

Study Author, Year PMID	Intervention (Control)	%Antiarrhythmic drug Class I	%Antiarrhythmic drug Class III	%Beta blocker	%ACEi or ARB	Control (Verbatim)
		Medications Intervention (Control)				
ICD vs. no ICD						
AMIOVIRT Strickberger, 2003 12767651	ICD (Amiodarone)	nd	Amiodarone: 0 (100)	Last follow-up: 53 (50)	Last follow-up: 90 (81)	Subjects were randomly assigned to receive either amiodarone or an ICD.
CABG-Patch Bigger, 1997 9371853	ICD (No ICD)	17 (12)	Amiodarone: 4 (3); Sotalol: 1 (0.2)	18 (24)	ACEi: 55 (54)	Patients were randomly assigned to the defibrillator or control group within randomly permuted blocks. The trial protocol prohibited the use of antiarrhythmic drugs for asymptomatic ventricular arrhythmia and specified that patients without contraindications should be treated with aspirin.
CAT Bansch, 2002 11914254	ICD (Control)	nd	nd	4 (4)	ACEi: 94 (98)	Patients with recent onset of DCM (9 months) and an ejection fraction 30% were randomly assigned to the implantation of an ICD or control.
Chan, 2009 20031808	ICD (No ICD)	1 (0.4)	Class III: 8 (8)	86 (83)	86 (86)	The study cohort comprised 965 patients (751 [77.8%] ischemic; 214 [22.2%] nonischemic), of whom 494 (51.2%) received ICDs.
COMPANION Bristow, 2004 15152059	ICD + CRT (No ICD)	nd	nd	68 (66)	90 (89)	Eligible patients who provided written informed consent were randomly assigned in a 1:2:2 ratio to treatment with protocol-mandated optimal pharmacologic therapy alone, optimal pharmacologic therapy plus cardiac-resynchronization therapy with a pacemaker, or optimal pharmacologic therapy plus cardiac-resynchronization therapy with a pacemaker–defibrillator. The pharmacologic therapy used in all groups consisted of diuretics (unless they were not needed), ACEi (unless they were not tolerated, where-upon ARBs could be substituted), beta-blockers (unless they were not tolerated or were contraindicated), and spironolactone (unless it was not tolerated). Digoxin and other medications used to treat heart failure could be given at the investigator's discretion.

Study Author, Year PMID	Intervention (Control)	Medications Intervention (Control)		%Beta blocker	%ACEi or ARB	Control (Verbatim)
		%Antiarrhythmic drug Class I	%Antiarrhythmic drug Class III			
DEFINITE Kadish, 2004 15152060	ICD (No ICD)	nd	Amiodarone: 4 (7)	86 (84)	ACEi: 84 (87); ARB: 14 (9)	Patients were randomly assigned to receive either standard oral medical therapy for heart failure or standard oral medical therapy plus an ICD. All patients received ACEi unless they were contraindicated. Patients who were unable to tolerate ACE inhibitors received hydralazine or nitrates or ARBs. In addition, beta-blocker therapy was required unless patients were unable to tolerate it. Carvedilol was the beta-blocker of choice on the basis of data available when the study was designed. The doses of ACEi and beta-blockers were adjusted to the levels recommended for patients with heart failure or to the highest tolerated doses. Digoxin and diuretics were used when necessary to manage clinical symptoms. The use of antiarrhythmic drugs such as amiodarone was discouraged. However, it was recognized that some patients had symptomatic atrial fibrillation or supraventricular arrhythmias requiring treatment with amiodarone, and these conditions did not constitute exclusion criteria. No other antiarrhythmic drugs were used.
DINAMIT Hohnloser, 2004 15590950	ICD (No ICD)	nd	nd	87 (87)	95 (94)	Patients were randomly assigned in a 1:1 ratio either to receive an ICD (the ICD group) or not to receive an ICD (the control group). The study protocol mandated that patients receive the best conventional medical therapy. Investigators were encouraged to treat all study patients with ACEi, beta-blockers, aspirin, and lipid-lowering drugs, as appropriate.
Fonarow, 2000 10760339	ICD (Control)	4 (12)	Amiodarone: 40 (36)	0 (5)	ACEi: 83 (74)	Of the 147 patients, 122 were treated with conventional medical therapy. Patients with atrial fibrillation or frequent nonsustained VT received low-dose amiodarone (200 mg/day) after varied loading protocols. Type I antiarrhythmic agents for nonsustained VT or atrial fibrillation were generally discontinued.

Study Author, Year PMID	Intervention (Control)	Medications Intervention (Control) %Antiarrhythmic drug Class I	%Antiarrhythmic drug Class III	%Beta blocker	%ACEi or ARB	Control (Verbatim)
IRIS Steinbeck, 2009 19812399	ICD (No ICD)	"Anti-arrhythmic drugs (mainly amiodarone): 13 (17)	"Anti-arrhythmic drugs (mainly amiodarone): 13 (17)	89 (86)	82 (82)	The remaining 898 patients (86% of whom were still in the hospital) were randomly assigned to a study treatment — 445 to receive an ICD and 453 to receive medical therapy alone — at a mean (±SD) of 13±7 days after infarction.
MADIT Moss, 1996 8960472	ICD (No ICD)	At 1 mo: 12 (10)	At 1 mo: Amiodarone: 2 (74); Sotalol: 1 (7); Sotalol and beta-blockers: 27 (15)	At 1 mo: 26 (8)	At 1 mo: ACEi: 60 (55)	The choice of conventional medical therapy, including the decision whether to use antiarrhythmic medications, was left to the patient's attending physician. Antiarrhythmic drugs approved and released by the FDA could be administered to patients in either group.
MADIT II Moss, 2002 11907286	ICD (No ICD)	3 (2)	Amiodarone: 13 (10)	70 (70)	ACEi: 68 (72)	The patients were randomly assigned in a 3:2 ratio to receive either an implantable defibrillator or conventional medical therapy. The appropriate use of beta-blockers, ACEi, and lipid-lowering drugs was strongly encouraged in both study groups.
Mezu, 2011 21640321	ICD (No ICD)	I and III: 9 (22)	I and III: 9 (22)	70 (61)	ACEi: 77 (65)	We identified all patients who received an ICD at our institution from January 2000 through December 2008 and were 80 years of age at the time of their ICD implantation.
OPTIMIZE-HF and GWTG-HF Hernandez, 2010 20009044	ICD (No ICD)	nd	nd	84 (78)	78 (72)	We identified patients with heart failure who were aged 65 years or older and were eligible for an ICD, had left ventricular ejection fraction of 35% or less, and were discharged alive from hospitals participating in the Organized Program to Initiate Lifesaving Treatment in Hospitalized Patients With Heart Failure and the Get With the Guidelines–Heart Failure quality-improvement programs during the period January 1, 2003, through December 31, 2006. We matched the patients to Medicare claims to examine long-term outcomes.
SCD-HeFT Bardy, 2005 15659722	ICD (No ICD/placebo)	nd	nd	At enrollment: 69 (69)	At enrollment: 94 (97)	From September 16, 1997, to July 18, 2001, we randomly assigned 2521 patients in equal proportions to receive placebo, amiodarone, or a single-chamber ICD programmed to shock-only mode.
ICD vs. CRT-D						
Diab, 2011 21700757	ICD (CRT-D)	nd	nd	73 (71)	100 (98)	All patients underwent a device implantation procedure but were blinded to whether they received a CRT-D or an ICD device.

Study Author, Year PMID	Intervention (Control)	Medications Intervention (Control)		%Beta blocker	%ACEi or ARB	Control (Verbatim)
		%Antiarrhythmic drug Class I	%Antiarrhythmic drug Class III			
MADIT-CRT Moss, 2009 19723701	ICD (CRT-D)	0.4 (1)	Amiodarone: 7 (7)	93 (93)	ACEi: 77 (77); ARB: 20 (21)	The patients were randomly assigned in a 3:2 ratio to receive either CRT with an ICD (CRT–ICD group) or only an ICD (ICD-only group) and were stratified according to clinical center and ischemic status with the use of an algorithm that ensured near balance in each stratum.
MENDMI Chung, 2010 20852059	ICD (CRT-D)	nd	nd	94 (94)	94 (88)	Eligible patients were randomized 1:1 in blocks of 4 stratified per center to therapy CRT-D or control (ICD) between 3 and 14 days of their presenting MI.
RAFT Tang, 2010 21073365	ICD (CRT-D)	nd	nd	89 (90)	97 (96)	Eligible patients were randomly assigned in a 1:1 ratio to receive an ICD or an ICD with CRT and were stratified according to clinical center, atrial rhythm (atrial fibrillation or flutter or sinus–atrial pacing), and a planned implantation of a single- or dual-chamber ICD.

ACEi=angiotensin-converting-enzyme inhibitor, ARB=angiotensin receptor blockers, CRT-D=cardiac resynchronization therapy defibrillator, ICD=implantable cardiac defibrillator, nd=not documented, VT=ventricular tachycardia

For study names, see Appendix Table 1.

Appendix Table 3. ICD vs. No ICD: Results for all-cause mortality at longest follow-up

Study Author, Year PMID	Outcome name	Timepoint	Outcome description	Intervention (Control)	Events Intervention (Control)	N analyzed Intervention (Control)	Metric	Results (95% CI)	p-value between arms
≥4 year									
MADIT II Barsheshet, 2011 210448997	Death, all-cause longest follow-up	8 y	nd	ICD (No ICD)	~44%[1] (~55%)	567 (490)	Adjusted HR	0.55 (0.46-0.67)	<0.001
CAT Bansch, 2002 11914254	Death, all-cause longest follow-up	5 y	nd	ICD (No ICD)	13 (17)	50 (54)	nd	nd	nd
DEFINITE Kadish, 2004 15152060	Death, all-cause longest follow-up	5 y	nd	ICD (No ICD)	28 (40)	229 (229)	Unadjusted HR[2]	0.65 (0.40-1.06)	0.08
MADIT Moss, 1996 8960472	Death, all-cause longest follow-up	5 y	nd	ICD (No ICD)	15 (39)	95 (101)	HR	0.46 (0.26-0.82)	0.009
SCD-HeFT Bardy, 2005 15659722	Death, all-cause longest follow-up	5 y	nd	ICD (No ICD/placebo)	182 (240)	829 (845)	nd	nd	nd
MADIT II Moss, 2002 11907286	Death, all-cause longest follow-up	4 y	nd	ICD (No ICD)	105 (97)	742 (490)	HR	0.69 (0.51-0.93)	0.016
2-3 y									
Chan, 2009 20031808	Death, all-cause longest follow-up	3 y	Death at 34 ± 16 mo in ICD arm; Death at 33 ± 16 mo in No ICD arm	ICD (No ICD)	102 (115)	494 (471)	Adjusted HR	0.69 (0.50-0.96)	0.03
OPTIMIZE-HF and GWTG-HF Hernandez, 2010 20009044	Death, all-cause longest follow-up	3 y	Death at 3 y	ICD (No ICD)	101 (1771)	376 (4,309)	Inverse-weighted HR (control for meds)	0.71 (0.56-0.91)[3]	<0.001

1 Estimated from figure
2 Adjusted model "unchanged" at 0.65 but CI not reported
3 Unadjusted HR 0.67 (0.52-0.87)

Study Author, Year PMID	Outcome name	Timepoint	Outcome description	Intervention (Control)	Events Intervention (Control)	N analyzed Intervention (Control)	Metric	Results (95% CI)	p-value between arms
AMIOVIRT Strickberger, 2003 12767651	Death, all-cause longest follow-up	2 y	Duration of follow-up 2.2 y ion ICD arm and 1.8 y in Amiodarone arm	ICD (Amiodarone)	6 (7)	51 (52)	nd	nd	0.8
DEFINITE Kadish, 2004 15152060	Death, all-cause longest follow-up	2 y	nd	ICD (No ICD)	7.9% (14.1%)	229 (229)	nd	nd	nd
Fonarow, 2000 10760339	Death, all-cause longest follow-up	2 y	nd	ICD (No ICD)	2 (31)	25 (122)	nd	nd	nd
MADIT II Moss, 2002 11907286	Death, all-cause longest follow-up	2 y	nd	ICD (No ICD)	~15%[4] (~31%)	742 (490)	% difference	-28% (-46%, 4%)	NS
Mezu, 2011 21640321	Death, all-cause longest follow-up	2 y	Death during study	ICD (No ICD)	58 (35)	99 (53)	nd	nd	nd
OPTIMIZE-HF and GWTG-HF Hernandez, 2010 20009044	Death, all-cause longest follow-up	2 y	Death at 2 y	ICD (No ICD)	90 (1550)	376 (4,309)	nd	nd	<0.001
CABG-Patch Bigger, 1997 9371853	Death, all-cause longest follow-up	3 y	Death at 32 ± 16 mo	ICD (No ICD)	101 (95)	446 (454)	HR, Cox adjusted for 10 prespecified covariates	1.03 (0.75-1.41)	NS
DINAMIT Hohnloser, 2004 15590950	Death, all-cause longest follow-up	3 y	All cause mortality at 30 ± 13 mo	ICD (No ICD)	62 (58)	332 (342)	HR	1.08 (0.76-1.55)	0.66
IRIS Steinbeck, 2009 19812399	Death, all-cause longest follow-up	3 y	nd	ICD (No ICD)	116 (117)	445 (453)	HR	1.04 (0.81-1.35)	0.15
		2 y			15.4% (18.2%)	445 (453)	nd	nd	nd

4 Estimated from figure

1 y

Study Author, Year PMID	Outcome name	Timepoint	Outcome description	Intervention (Control)	Events Intervention (Control)	N analyzed Intervention (Control)	Metric	Results (95% CI)	p-value between arms
AMIOVIRT Strickberger, 2003 12767651	Death, all-cause longest follow-up	1 y	nd	ICD (Amiodarone)	96% (90%)	51 (52)	nd	nd	nd
CAT Bansch, 2002 11914254	Death, all-cause longest follow-up	1 y	nd	ICD (No ICD)	4 (2)	50 (54)	nd	nd	nd
COMPANION Bristow, 2004 15152059	Death, all-cause longest follow-up	1 y	Death from any cause	ICD + CRT (No ICD)	105 (77)	595 (308)	HR	0.76 (0.58-1.01)	0.059 (Adjusted 0.06)
DEFINITE Kadish, 2004 15152060	Death, all-cause longest follow-up	1 y	nd	ICD (No ICD)	2.6% (6.2%)	229 (229)	nd	nd	nd
Fonarow, 2000 10760339	Death, all-cause longest follow-up	1 y	nd	ICD (Control)	6.7% (24.5%)	25 (122)	nd	nd	nd
MADIT II Moss, 2002 11907286	Death, all-cause longest follow-up	1 y	nd	ICD (No ICD)	~8%[5] (~10%)	742 (490)	% difference	-12% (-40%, 27%)	NS
Mezu, 2011 21640321	Death, all-cause longest follow-up	1 y	Death at 1 y	ICD (No ICD)	72% (52%)	99 (53)	Adjusted HR[6]	0.78 (0.44-1.30)	0.312
OPTIMIZE-HF and GWTG-HF Hernandez, 2010 20009044	Death, all-cause longest follow-up	1 y	Death at 1 y	ICD (No ICD)	65 (1102)	376 (4,309)	nd	nd	<0.001
IRIS Steinbeck, 2009 19812399	Death, all-cause longest follow-up	1 y	nd	ICD (No ICD)	10.6% (12.5%)	445 (453)	nd	nd	nd

CI=confidence interval, HR=hazards ratio, ICD=implantable cardiac defibrillator, mo=month, nd=not documented, NS=not significant, y=year
For study names, see Appendix Table 1.

[5] Estimated from figure
[6] Adjusted for age, Charlson comorbidity index, LVEF, GFR

Appendix Table 4. ICD plus CRT versus ICD alone: Results for all-cause mortality at longest followup

Study Author, Year PMID	Outcome name	Timepoint	Outcome description	Intervention (Control)	Events Intervention (Control)	N analyzed Intervention (Control)	Metric	Results (95% CI)	p-value between arms
≥4 year									
MADIT-CRT Moss, 2009 19723701	Death, all-cause longest followup	5 y	nd	CRT-D (ICD)	74 (53)	nd	HR	1.00 (0.69-1.44)	0.99
3 years									
RAFT Tang, 2010 21073365	Death, all-cause longest followup	3 y	Death from any cause	CRT-D (ICD)	186 (236)	894 (904)	HR	0.75 (0.62-0.91)	0.003
1 y									
Diab, 2011 21700757	Death, all-cause longest followup	1 y	Mortality	CRT-D (ICD)	0 (2)	nd	nd	nd	nd
MENDMI Chung 2010 20852059	Death, all-cause longest followup	1 y	All-cause mortality	CRT-D (ICD)	1 (1)	42 (38)	nd	nd	1.00

CI=confidence interval, CRT-D=cardiac resynchronization therapy defibrillator, HR=hazards ratio, nd=not documented, y=year

For study names, see Appendix Table 1.

Appendix Table 5. Subgroup analyses of ICD vs. no ICD for all-cause death

Study, Author, Year, PMID	Subgroups HR/RR	(95% CI)	P Interaction
Age			
MADIT, Moss, 1996, 8960472	Continuous: nd		P>0.2
CABG-Patch, Bigger, 1997, 9371853	Continuous: nd		NS
MADIT II, Moss, 2002, 11907286	<60 y: 0.5 (0.2, 0.9) ≥70 y: 0.6 (0.45, 0.95)	60-69 y: 0.8 (0.5, 1.3)	NS
DINAMIT, Hohnloser, 2004, 15590950	<60 y: 0.9 (0.4, 1.9)	≥60 y: 1.2 (0.8, 1.9)	P=0.46
Chan, 2009, 20031808*	<65 y: 0.74 (0.43,1.28) ≥75 y: 0.59 (0.39, 0.90)	65-74 y: 0.76 (0.45, 1.29)	P=0.43
COMPANION, Bristow, 2004, 15152059	≤65 y: 0.6 (0.3, 0.95)	>65 y: 0.7 (0.5, 1.0)	nd
SCD-HeFT, Bardy 2005 15659722	<65 y: 0.68 (0.50, 0.93)†	≥65 y: 0.86 (0.62, 1.18)†	nd
DEFINITE, Kadish, 2004, 15152060	<65y: 0.7 (0.3, 1.4)	≥65 y: 0.6 (0.3, 1.2)	NS
IRIS, Steinbeck, 2009, 19812399	<65 y: 0.95 (0.6, 1.5)	≥65 y: 1.05 (0.8, 1.5)	P=0.73
OPTIMIZE-HF and GWTG-H, Hernandez, 2010, 20009044*	65-74 y: 0.65 (0.47, 0.89)	75-84 y: 0.80 (0.62, 1.03)	P=0.31
Sex			
CABG-Patch, Bigger, 1997, 9371853	Female: nd	Male: nd	NS
COMPANION, Bristow, 2004, 15152059	0.6 (0.3, 1.1)	0.65 (0.4, 0.9)	nd
DEFINITE, Kadish, 2004, 15152060	1.1 (0.5-2.6)	0.49 (0.27, 0.90)	NS
DINAMIT, Hohnloser, 2004, 15590950	1.0 (0.5-2.1)	1.1 (0.7-1.7)	P=0.82
IRIS, Steinbeck, 2009, 19812399	1.0 (0.6-1.7)	1.1 (0.8-1.5)	P=0.85
MADIT II Moss, 2002, 11907286	0.6 (0.3-1.1)	0.7 (0.5-0.9)	NS
MADIT, Moss, 1996, 8960472	nd	nd	P>0.2
OPTIMIZE-HF and GWTG-H, Hernandez, 2010, 20009044*	0.58 (0.41,0.83)	0.80 (0.63,1.01)	P=0.15
SCD-HeFT, Russo 2008 18373605	0.90 (0.56, 1.43)†	0.71 (0.57, 0.88)†	P=0.54‡
Race/Ethnicity			
SCD-HeFT, Mitchell, 2008, 18294487	AA: 0.65 (0.43, 0.99)†	White: 0.73 (0.58, 0.90)†	P=0.53
Bardy 2005 15659722	Non-white: 0.75 (0.48, 1.17)†	White: 0.78 (0.61, 1.00)†	nd
NYHA Class			
CABG-Patch, Bigger, 1997, 9371853	nd		NS
COMPANION, Bristow, 2004, 15152059	III: 0.6 (0.4, 0.97)	IV: 0.6 (0.4, 1.0)	nd
DEFINITE, Kadish, 2004, 15152060	I: 0.5 (0.2, 1.5) III: 0.37 (0.15, 0.90)	II: 1.0 (0.5, 2.2)	NS
DINAMIT, Hohnloser, 2004, 15590950	0-II: 1.1 (0.7, 1.7)	III: 1.0 (0.5, 2.3)	P=0.87
MADIT, Moss, 1996, 8960472	nd		P>0.2
MADIT II Moss, 2002, 11907286	I 0.6 (0.5, 0.9)	II-IV: 0.7 (0.45, 1.0)	NS
SCD-HeFT, Bardy 2005 15659722	II: 0.54 (0.40, 0.74)†	III: 1.16 (0.84, 1.61)†	**P<0.001**

Study, Author, Year, PMID	Subgroups HR/RR	(95% CI)			P Interaction
Heart Failure					
CABG-Patch, Bigger, 1997, 9371853	Yes:	nd	No:	nd	NS
Chan, 2009, 20031808*		0.69 (0.50, 0.93)		0.70 (0.35, 1.41)	P=0.59
MADIT, Moss, 1996, 8960472		nd		nd	P>0.2
IRIS, Steinbeck, 2009, 19812399		1.0 (0.7, 1.4)		1.2 (0.8, 1.8)	P=0.56
Time Since Heart Failure Diagnosis					
DEFINITE, Kadish, 2006, 16781376	≤3 mo:	0.38 (0.14, 1.000)	>3 mo:	0.80 (0.46,1.41)	P=0.19
	≤9 mo:	0.46 (0.216, 0.986)	>9 mo:	0.86 (0.46,1.61)	P=0.22
LVEF					
CABG-Patch, Bigger, 1997, 9371853		nd			NS
Chan, 2009, 20031808*	≤25%:	0.73 (0.51, 1.04)	26-35%:	0.59 (0.37, 0.93)	P=0.61
COMPANION, Bristow, 2004, 15152059	≤20:	0.6 (0.4, 0.9)	20-35%:	0.7 (0.4, 1.1)	nd
DEFINITE, Kadish, 2004, 15152060	<20%:	0.9 (0.4, 2.0)	20-36%:	0.5 (0.3,0.95)	NS
DINAMIT, Hohnloser, 2004, 15590950	<26%:	1.5 (0.8, 2.7)	26-35%:	0.85 (0.5, 1.5)	P=0.16
OPTIMIZE-HF and GWTG-H, Hernandez, 2010, 20009044*	≤30%:	0.76 (0.59, 0.98)§	All patients:	0.71 (0.56, 0.91)§	NA
MADIT, Moss, 1996, 8960472	Continuous:	nd			P>0.2
MADIT II, Moss, 2002, 11907286	≤25%:	0.6 (0.5, 0.9)	25-30%:	0.7 (0.4, 1.2)	NS
SCD-HeFT, Bardy 2005 15659722	≤30%:	0.73 (0.57, 0.92)†	30-35%:	1.08 (0.57, 2.07)†	nd
LBBB					
COMPANION, Bristow, 2004, 15152059	LBBB:	0.5 (0.4, 0.8)	Other:	0.9 (0.5, 1.6)	nd
MADIT, Moss, 1996, 8960472	LBBB:	nd	No LBBB:	nd	P>0.2
MADIT II, Moss, 2002, 11907286	LBBB:	nd	No LBBB:	nd	NS
QRS Duration					
CABG-Patch, Bigger, 1997, 9371853	≤100 msec:	nd	>100 msec:	nd	NS
COMPANION, Bristow, 2004, 15152059	≤147 msec:	0.8 (0.4, 1.3)	148-168 msec:	0.6 (0.3, 1.0)	nd
	>168 msec:	0.5 (0.3, 0.97)			
DEFINITE, Kadish, 2004, 15152060	<120 msec:	0.75 (0.4, 1.5)	≥120 msec:	0.5 (0.2, 1.1)	NS
DINAMIT, Hohnloser, 2004, 15590950	<120 msec:	0.85 (0.5, 1.4)	≥120 msec:	1.5 (0.8, 2.9)	P=0.13
MADIT II, Moss, 2002, 11907286	<120 msec:	0.7 (0.5, 1.2)	120-150 msec:	0.6 (0.4, 1.1)	NS
	≥150 msec:	0.5 (0.3, 0.9)			
SCD-HeFT, Bardy 2005 15659722	<120 msec:	0.84 (0.62, 1.14)†	≥120 msec:	0.67 (0.49, 0.93)†	nd
Heart Disease					
COMPANION, Bristow, 2004, 15152059	Ischemic:	0.73 (0.52, 1.04)	Non-ischemic:	0.5 (0.29, 0.88)	NS
Time Since Myocardial Infarction					
SCD-HeFT, Piccini, 2011, 21109025	<18 mo:	0.7 (0.37, 1.31)†	18-51 mo:	0.54 (0.3, 0.98)†	P=0.33
	52-111 mo:	1.47 (0.75, 2.87)†	>111 mo:	0.75 (0.44, 1.29)†	
MADIT, Moss, 1996, 8960472	<6 mo:	nd	≥6 mo:	nd	P>0.2
MADIT II, Moss, 2002, 11907286	<6 mo:	nd	≥6 mo:	nd	NS

Study, Author, Year, PMID	Subgroups HR/RR	(95% CI)	P Interaction
MADIT II, Wilber, 2004, 14993128	<18 mo: 0.97 (0.51, 1.81)	≥18 mo: 0.55 (0.39, 0.78)	P=0.27
	18-59 mo 0.52 (0.26, 1.05)	60-119 mo 0.50 (0.26, 0.91)	nd
	≥120 mo: 0.62 (0.36, 1.08)		
Prior Coronary Revasc			
MADIT, Moss, 1996, 8960472	CR: nd	No CR: nd	P>0.2
SCD-HeFT, Al-Khatib 2008 18479330	CABG: 0.87 (0.62, 1.22)	No CABG: 0.66 (0.47, 0.94)	P=0.39
	PCI: 0.66 (0.36, 1.22)	No PCI: 0.82 (0.53, 1.29)	P=0.93
Time Since Coronary Revasc			
MADIT II, Goldenberg, 2006, 16682305	≤6 mo: 1.19 (0.40, 3.54)	>6 mo: 0.64 (0.45, 0.90)	P=0.29
	7-60 mo: 0.55 (0.31, 0.97)	>60 mo 0.67 (0.43, 1.03)	nd
SCD-HeFT, Al-Khatib 2008 18479330	CABG ≤2 y: 1.40 (0.61, 3.24)	CABG >2 y: 0.71 (0.49, 1.04)	P=0.09
	Time since PCI: nd		P=0.51
Diabetes Mellitus			
CABG-Patch, Bigger, 1997, 9371853	Yes: nd	No: nd	NS
Chan, 2009, 20031808*	0.68 (0.45, 1.03)	0.69 (0.48, 1.01)	P=0.95
DINAMIT, Hohnloser, 2004, 15590950	0.9 (0.5, 1.5)	1.2 (0.8, 2.0)	P=0.38
IRIS, Steinbeck, 2009, 19812399	nd	nd	NS
MADIT II, Moss, 2002, 11907286	nd	nd	NS
SCD-HeFT, Bardy 2005 15659722	0.95 (0.68, 1.33)†	0.67 (0.50, 0.90)†	nd
Blood Urea Nitrogen			
MADIT, Moss, 1996, 8960472	≤25 mg/dL: nd	>25 mg/dL: nd	P>0.2
MADIT II Moss, 2002, 11907286	≤25 mg/dL: nd	>25 mg/dL: nd	NS
Kidney Disease			
Chan, 2009, 20031808*	Kidney failure: 0.52 (0.11, 2.48)	No kidney failure: 0.70 (0.53, 0.94)	P=0.21
MADIT II, Goldenberg, 2006, 16893702	eGFR ≥35: 1.09 (0.49, 2.43)	eGFR <35: 0.68 (0.50, 0.93)	P=0.29
	eGFR 35-59: 0.74 (0.48, 1.15)	eGFR ≥60: 0.66 (0.43, 1.02)	nd

AA = African American, CABG = coronary artery bypass graft, CI =confidence interval, CR = coronary revascularization, eGFR = estimated glomerular filtration rate (in mL/min/m^2), HR = hazard ratio, ICD = implantable cardiac defibrillator, LBBB = left bundle branch block, LVEF = left ventricular ejection fraction, mo = month, NA = not applicable, nd =no data, NS = Not statistically significant (no P-value documented), PCI = percutaneous coronary revascularization, PMID = PubMed ID, Revasc = revascularization, RR = risk ratio, y = years. See page 16 for study acronyms

* Nonrandomized comparative study

† 97.5% confidence interval

‡ P value refers to comparison of subgroups across all three study arms. (ICD, amiodarone, and placebo).

§ Only the LVEF <30% subgroup analysis was reported. The alternative group given here is from the total analysis, regardless of LVEF.

Appendix Table 6. ICD vs. No ICD: Results for 30 d mortality

Study Author, Year PMID	Outcome name	Timepoint	Outcome description	Intervention (Control)	Events Intervention (Control)	N analyzed Intervention (Control)	Metric	Results (95% CI)	p-value between arms
CABG-Patch Bigger, 1997 9371853	Death, all-cause at 30 d	30 d	Death in the first 30 days	ICD (No ICD)	24 (20)	446 (454)	nd	nd	0.60
MADIT Moss, 1996 8960472	Death, all-cause at 30 d	30 d	NR	ICD (No ICD)	0 (0)	95 (101)	nd	nd	nd

CI=confidence interval, d= day, ICD=implantable cardiac defibrillator, nd=not documented

Appendix Table 7. ICD vs. No ICD: Results for sudden cardiac (arrhythmic) death

Study Author, Year PMID	Outcome name	Timepoint	Outcome description	Intervention (Control)	Events Intervention (Control)	N analyzed Intervention (Control)	Metric	Results (95% CI)	p-value between arms
5 y									
MADIT Moss, 1996 8960472	Death, cardiac arrhythmia	5 y	Classification of Hinkle and Thaler 13 was used to evaluate the suspected mechanism of death from cardiac causes (arrhythmic or nonarrhythmic). "Abrupt loss of consciousness and disappearance of pulse without prior collapse of the circulation" (w/ or w/o CHF; witnessed or not)	ICD (No ICD)	3 (13)	95 (101)	nd	nd	nd
3 y									
Chan, 2009 20031808	Death, cardiac arrhythmia	3 y	Death arrhythmic, Modified Hinkle and Thaler: unwitnessed deaths (if stable when last observed within 24 hours before death), witnessed instantaneous deaths, and sequelae of cardiac arrest.	ICD (No ICD)	46 (105)	494 (471)	Adjusted HR	0.65 (0.40-1.03)	0.07
DINAMIT Hohnloser, 2004 15590950	Death, cardiac arrhythmia	3 y	Death due to cardiac arrhythmia from witnesses, family, death certificate, hospital records, autopsy. Not ICD telemetry	ICD (No ICD)	12 (29)	332 (342)	HR	0.42 (0.22-0.83)	0.009
IRIS Steinbeck, 2009 19812399	Death, cardiac arrhythmia	3 y	A death, either in the hospital or out of the hospital, was assumed to be a sudden cardiac death if a cardiac death occurred within minutes after the onset of acute symptoms, resulted from a documented cardiac arrhythmia, or was not witnessed and occurred unexpectedly and without recognizable causes (e.g., during sleep). Furthermore, a death was classified as a sudden cardiac death regardless of the underlying condition.	ICD (No ICD)	27 (60)	445 (453)	HR	0.55 (0.31-1.00)	0.049
2 y									
AMIOVIRT Strickberger, 2003 12767651	Death, cardiac arrhythmia	2 y	Sudden cardiac death (actual death); Cardiac death, SCD, duration of follow up 2.2 y	ICD (Amiodarone)	1 (2)	51 (52)	nd	nd	0.7
DEFINITE Kadish, 2004 15152060	Death, cardiac arrhythmia	2 y	Sudden death from arrhythmia	ICD (No ICD)	3 (14)	229 (229)	HR	0.20 (0. 60-0.71)	0.001

TA on ICD for Primary Prevention
Appendix C

Study Author, Year PMID	Outcome name	Timepoint	Outcome description	Intervention (Control)	Events Intervention (Control)	N analyzed Intervention (Control)	Metric	Results (95% CI)	p-value between arms
Fonarow, 2000 10760339	Death, cardiac arrhythmia	2 y	Witnessed cardiac arrest or death within at least 1 hour after onset of acute symptoms or unexpected, unwitnessed death in a patient known to have been well within the previous 24 hours	ICD (Control)	0 (18)	25 (122)	nd	nd	0.05
			Actuarial survival	ICD (Control)	100% (78.3%)	25 (122)	nd	nd	0.05
1 y									
CAT Bansch, 2002 11914254	Death, all-cause longest follow-up	1 y	Sudden cardiac death	ICD (No ICD)	0 (0)	50 (54)	nd	nd	nd

CHF=chronic heart failure, CI=confidence interval, CRT-D=cardiac resynchronization therapy defibrillator, HR=hazards ratio, ICD=implantable cardiac defibrillator, mo=month, nd=not documented, y=year

For study names, see Appendix Table 1.

C-17

Appendix Table 8. Risk of bias

Study Author, Year PMID	Overall	Random'n	Alloc Conc	Blinding	Attr'n	ITT	Base Similar	Coint'n	Other Factors	Crossover to ICD	Crossover to no ICD
ICD vs. no ICD											
AMIOVIRT Strickberger, 2003 12767651	Good	Low	Unclear	Low	Low	Low	Low	Low	Yes, highly underpowered	8/52 (15%)	3/51 (6%) heart transplants; 11/51 (22%) also started amiodarone
CABG-Patch Bigger, 1997 9371853	Fair[7]	Low	Low	High	Low	Low	Low	Low	Yes, differential crossover	18/454 (4%)	52/446 (12%)
CAT Bansch, 2002 11914254	Good	Low	Low	Unclear	Low	Low	Low	Low	Yes, highly underpowered	nd	nd
Chan, 2009 20031808	--	--	--	--	--	--	--	--	Yes, observational study	77/456 (17%)	nd
COMPANION Bristow, 2004 15152059	Fair	Low (implied)	Unclear	High	High	Low	Low	Low	Yes, differential attrition and crossover (patients censored when crossed over)	26%	6.5%
DEFINITE Kadish, 2004 15152060	Fair	Low	Unclear	Low	Low	Low	Low	Low	Yes, differential crossover	23/229 (10%)	4/229 (2%)
DINAMIT Hohnloser, 2004 15590950	Good	Low	Low	Low	Low	Low	Low	Low	No	nd	22/332 (7%)
Fonarow, 2000 10760339	--	--	--	--	--	--	--	--	Yes, observational study	0/122 (0%)	1/25 (4%)
IRIS Steinbeck, 2009 19812399	Good	Low (implied)	Unclear	Low	Low	Low	Low	Low	No	39/463 (8%)	45/445 (10%)
MADIT Moss, 1996 8960472	Good	Low	Unclear	Unclear	Low (14%)	Low	Low	Low	No	11/101 (11%)	7/95 (7%)
MADIT II Moss, 2002 11907286	Good[8]	Low (implied)	Unclear	High	Low	Low	Low	Low	No	22/490 (4%)	44/742 (6%)

---

[7] Poor outcome other than all-cause mortality

Study Author, Year PMID	Overall	Random'n	Alloc Conc	Blinding	Attr'n	ITT	Base Similar	Coint'n	Other Factors	Crossover to ICD	Crossover to no ICD
Mezu, 2011 21640321	--	--	--	--	--	--	--	--	Yes, observational study	nd	nd
OPTIMIZE-HF and GWTG-HF Hernandez, 2010 20009044	--	--	--	--	--	--	--	--	Yes, observational study	nd	nd
SCD-HeFT Bardy, 2005 15659722	Fair	Low (implied)	Unclear	Unclear	Low	Low	Low	High	Yes, differential crossover; differential use of beta blockers[9]	118/1676 (11%)	50/829 (6%)
ICD vs. CRT-D											
Diab, 2011 21700757	Good	Low	Low	Low	Low	Low	Low	Low	Yes, powered for echo outcomes	nd	nd
MADIT-CRT Moss, 2009 19723701	Good	Low (implied)	Unclear	Low	Low	Low	Low	Low	No	ICD→CRT 91/731 (12%); CRT→ICD 82/1089 (8%)	30/1820 (2%)
MENDMI Chung, 2010 20852059	Fair	Low (implied)	Unclear	Unclear	High	Low	Low	Low	Yes, powered for LVEDV	nd	nd
RAFT Tang, 2010 21073365	Good	Low	Unclear	Low	Low	Low	Low	Low	Yes, powered for the primary outcome, a composite of death or hospitalization for heart failure	nd	nd

Random'n: Randomization—What is the risk of selection bias (biased allocation to interventions) due to inadequate generation of a randomized sequence?

Alloc Conc: Allocation Concealment—What is the risk of selection bias (biased allocation to interventions) due to inadequate concealment of allocations before assignment?

Blinding: Outcome Assessor Blinding—For each main outcome or class of outcomes, what was the risk of detection bias due to knowledge of the allocated interventions by outcome assessment (lack of outcome assessor blinding)?

Attr'n: Attrition—For each main outcome or class of outcomes, what is the risk of attrition bias due to amount, nature, or handling of incomplete outcome data?

ITT: Intention-to-Treat—Were all randomized participants analyzed in the group to which they were allocated?

Base Similar: Groups Similarity—Were the groups similar at baseline regarding the most important prognostic indicators?

Coint'n: Cointerventions—Were co-interventions avoided or similar?

Other Factors: Are there other risks of bias? If yes, describe them in Notes?

Crossovers: Numbers of crossovers from one intervention to the other.

8 Fair outcomes other than all-cause mortality

9 Except in the use of beta-blockers at the time of the last follow-up visit (P<0.001). Amiodarone 72%; Placebo 79%; ICD 82%

nd=not documented

For study names, see Appendix Table 1.

Appendix Table 9. Quality of life in comparative studies of ICDs for primary prevention of SCD

Study Author, Year PMID	N	Study Duration	Intervention	QoL Instrument	Favors*	Net Difference†	95% CI†	Test Range "Worst"	"Best"	P Value
MADIT II Noyes, 2007 17446823	1,232	3 y	ICD vs. conventional treatment	Health Utility Index 3	0	-0.068	-	-0.371	1.0	NS
AMIOVIRT Strickberger, 2003 12767651	103	1 y	ICD vs. Amiodarone	Quality of Well-being Schedule	0	+7	-0.1, +14	0	110	NS
				State Trait Anxiety Inventory	0	-2	-10, +6	40	160	NS
CABG Patch Namerow, 1999 10527011	490	6 mo	ICD vs. control	SF-36: Physical Limitations	0	-7.5	-	0	100	NS
				Role - Physical	0	-3.5	-	0	100	NS
				Bodily Pain	0	-1.4	-	0	100	NS
				General Health	0	-3.5	-	0	100	NS
				Social Limitations	0	-0.3	-	0	100	NS
				Role - Emotional	No ICD	-11.9	-	0	100	0.003
				Mental Health	No ICD	-4.7	-	0	100	0.004
				Perception of Health Transition	No ICD	+0.3	-	5	1	0.030

CABG Patch= Coronary Artery Bypass Graft Patch; CI=confidence interval; HRQOL=health-related quality of life; ICD=implantable cardioverter-defibrillator; MADIT II=Multicenter Automatic Defibrillator Implantation Trial II; mo=month; NS=not statistically significant; PMID=PubMed ID; QOL=quality of life; y=year

* Notes arm with statistically significantly better change in QOL
† (ΔQOL ICD arm – ΔQOL Treatment arm), data calculated

Health Utility Index (HUI3) "is a questionnaire that assesses HRQOL across 8 attributes: vision, hearing, speech, ambulation, dexterity, emotion, cognition, and pain and discomfort and can take values between -0.371 and 1, with -0.371 being the worst possible health state, 0 being death, and 1 being the best possible health state." PMID 17446823

Perception of Health Transition Patients assess their current health status relative to 1 year before. Higher scores represent the perception that health status has gotten worse. PMID 10527011

Quality of Well-being Schedule "A higher level of general well-being is associated with a greater value." The score range is 0 to 110. PMID 12767651

SF-36 "The Medical Outcomes Study 36-Item Short-Form health survey is a widely used health status questionnaire comprised of 36 items... The SF-36 health survey taps 8 health concepts: physical functioning, role limitations due to physical problems, bodily pain, general health perceptions, vitality, social functioning, role limitations due to emotional problems, mental health, health transition (perceived change in health)." PMID 10747763

State Trait Anxiety Inventory (STAI) "The score range is 40 to 160. A greater value is associated with a lower level of anxiety." [PMID 12767651] The scale and direction of this scale is different from other reports using STAI.

Appendix Table 10. Relationship between shocks and quality of life in patients with ICDs for primary prevention of SCD

Study Author, Year PMID	N	Study Duration	Comparison	% With Any Shock	QoL Instrument		Favors*	Net Difference†	Test "Worst"	Range "Best"	P Value
MADIT-II Noyes, 2009 19929037	983	3 y	Shock (with ICD) vs. no shock (with or without ICD)	nd	Health Utility Index 3		No shocks	-0.044 adjusted ‡	-0.371	1.0	0.037
CABG Patch Namerow, 1999 10527011	262	6 mo	Shock vs. no shock (all with ICD)	38.5%	SF-36:	Physical Limitations	0	-8.0	0	100	NS
						Physical Functioning	0	-8.3	0	100	NS
						Bodily Pain	0	-1.0	0	100	NS
						General Health	0	-4.5	0	100	NS
						Social Functioning	0	-2.8	0	100	NS
						Role Emotional	0	-10.4	0	100	NS
						Mental Health	0	-3.0	0	100	NS
						Perception of Health Transition	0	+0.2	5	1	NS

CABG Patch= Coronary Artery Bypass Graft Patch; ICD=implantable cardioverter–defibrillator; MADIT II=Multicenter Automatic Defibrillator Implantation Trial II; mo=month; NS=not statistically significant; PMID=PubMed ID; QOL: quality of life; y: year.

* Notes whether shocks or no shocks have a statistically significant association with better QOL.

† (ΔQOL ICD arm – ΔQOL Treatment arm)

‡ Effect size of ICD shock since last HRQOL assessment (at 3, 12, 24 and 36 mo after randomization) adjusted for clinical events and randomization to ICD vs. no ICD arm. On Health Utility Index 3 scale, 1 represents perfect health, 0 represents death, and negative values implies HRQOL worse than death.

Appendix Table 11. Quality of reporting for adverse events

Study, Author, Year, PubMed ID	Q1	Q1a	Q2	Q3	Q4	Q5	Q6*	Q7†	Q8
Comparative studies									
ADRIA, Sticherling, 2011, 21156772	Yes	Yes	Yes	Yes	nd	Yes	Yes	Yes	Yes‡
ALTITUDE, Saxon, 2010, 21098452	Yes	Yes	Yes	Yes	nd	Yes	Yes	Yes	No
MADIT-CRT Moss, 2009, 19723701 Moss, 2005, 16274414 (protocol)	No	--	--	Yes	nd	Yes	Yes	Yes	No
MADIT-RIT Moss, 2012, 23131066	Yes	Yes	Yes	Yes	nd	Yes	Yes	Yes	Yes
MENDMI, Chung, 2010, 20852059	Yes	No	Yes	Yes	nd	Yes	Yes	Yes	Yes‡
Morrison, 2011, 21737019	Yes	Yes	Yes	Yes	nd	Yes	Yes	Yes	Yes
RAFT, Tang, 2010, 21073395 Parkash, 2012, 23159551 Tang, 2009, 19102034 (protocol)	No	--	--	Yes	nd	Yes	Yes	Yes	Yes‡
RIGHT, Gold, 2012, 21978966	Yes	Yes	Yes	Yes	nd	Yes	Yes	Yes	Yes
ICD arms from RCTs									
MADIT II, Moss, 2002, 11907286 §	No	--	--	nd	nd	No	Yes	Yes	--
SCD-HeFT, Bardy, 2005, 15659722 Freudenberger, 2007, 17485579	No	--	--	Yes	nd	Yes	Yes	Yes	--
Cohort studies									
NCDR ICD Database, 11 papers ||	Yes	Yes	Yes	Yes	Yes	Yes	Yes	Yes	--
EPD-Vision 2009-2012, 5 papers ¶	Yes	Yes	Yes	Yes	nd	Yes	Yes	Yes	--
Birnie, 2012, 22311781	Yes	Yes	Yes	nd	nd	No	Yes	Yes	--
Bode, 2012, 22753865	Yes	Yes	Yes	nd	nd	Yes	Yes	Yes	--
Brullmann 2012, 22154315	No	--	--	Yes**	nd	Yes	Yes	Yes	--
Brumberg, 2012, 22519559	Yes	Yes	Yes	nd	nd	No	Yes	Yes	--
Charytan, 2011, 21664735	Yes	Yes	Yes	nd	nd	No	Yes	Yes	--
Cheung, 2012, 22923271	Yes	Yes	Yes	Yes	nd	Yes	Yes	Yes	--
Desai, 2010, 20403488	Yes	Yes	Yes	Yes	nd	Yes	Yes	Yes	--
Ditchl, 2011, 21678454	Yes	Yes	Yes	Yes	nd	Yes	Yes	Yes	--
Gradeus, 2003, 12914630	Yes	No	Yes	Yes	nd	Yes	Yes	Yes	--
Hauser, 2012, 22396584	Yes	Yes	Yes	Yes	nd	Yes	Yes	Yes	--
Landolina, 2011, 21576653	Yes	Yes	Yes	Yes	nd	Yes	Yes	Yes	--

Study, Author, Year, PubMed ID	Q1	Q1a	Q2	Q3	Q4	Q5	Q6*	Q7†	Q8
Larsen, 2010, 20186244	Yes	Yes	Yes	nd	nd	No	Yes	Yes	--
Lee, 2010 20170816; McFadden 2012, 22312139	Yes	Yes	Yes	Yes	nd	Yes	Yes	Yes	--
Lyman, 2011, 21795298	Yes	Yes	Yes	nd	nd	No	Yes	Yes	--
Kleeman, 2012, 22313314	Yes	Yes	Yes	Yes	nd	Yes	Yes	Yes	--
Porterfield, 2010, 19925609	Yes	Yes	Yes	nd	nd	Yes	Yes	Yes	--
Remmelts, 2009, 19325900	Yes	Yes	Yes	nd	nd	No	Yes	Yes	--
Sandesara, 2011, 21086086	Yes	Yes	Yes	Yes	nd	Yes	Yes	Yes	--
Schaer, 2011, 21712284	Yes	No	Yes	Yes	Yes	Yes	Yes	Yes	--
Sengupta, 2012, 22314669	No	--	--	nd	nd	No	Yes	Yes	--
Sweeney, 2012, 22387371	Yes	Yes	Yes	Yes	nd	Yes	No††	Yes	--
Sweeney, 2010, 21085109	Yes	No	Yes	Yes	nd	No	Yes	Yes	--
Sweeney, 2005, 15927965	Yes	Yes	Yes	Yes	nd	Yes	Yes	Yes	--
Tsai, 2010, 19262366	No	--	--	nd	nd	No	Yes	Yes	--
Tzogias, 2012, 22314669	Yes	Yes	Yes	nd	nd	No	Yes	Yes	--
Varma, 2010, 20716717	Yes	Yes	Yes	Yes	nd	Yes	Yes	Yes	--
Total Yes/Total	**31/38**	**27/31**	**27/27**	**26/38**	**2/38**	**27/38**	**37/38**	**38/38**	**6/8**

Modified McHarms
Q1. Were any harms prespecified (*a priori*) in Methods section?
Q1a. If yes, were any of them prespecified with *a priori* standardized or precise definitions?
Q2. Were all prespecified harms reported?
Q3. Was the mode of harms collection ACTIVE (sought to collect information on AEs)?
Q4. Was the mode of harms collection PASSIVE? (Participants are not specifically asked about or tested for the occurrence of adverse events. Rather, adverse events are identified based on patient reports made on their own initiative.)
Q5. Did the study specify the TIMING and/or FREQUENCY of collection of harms?
Q6. Is the number of participants who experience harms provided for each arm?
Q7. Is the number at risk for harms (denominator) provided for each arm?
Q8. For studies comparing adverse events across two or more arms: Is there a STATISTICAL analysis of relative harms between groups?

EPD-Vision=Cardiology Information System, Leiden University Medical Center; ICD=implantable cardioverter-defibrillator; NCDR: National Cardiovascular Data Registry; nd=not documented; RCT=randomized, controlled trial. For study name abbreviations, see Appendix Tables 1 and 16.
* Studies had to report number of patients affected.
† Studies had to report number of patients at risk.
‡ Not all outcomes
§ Additional information from protocol paper: Moss et al. *Annals of Noninvasive Electrocardiology* 1999. 4 (1): 83-91.

|| PMIDs: 22095828, 21878667, 21537001, 19383957, 21050975, 21867834, 20863954, 21487093, 19879533, 21883101 and 19221223

¶ PMIDs: 21208947, 19808497, 22056722, 22094073 and 21272746

** Active collection for inappropriate shocks. No data for other outcomes.

†† Number of patients affected not documented. Study used for subgroup table only.

Appendix Table 12. Early (in-hospital) adverse events from the NCDR ICD database - Study characteristics

Author, Year PMID	N	Primary Prevention	Dates	# Sites*	Exclusion Criteria (Prior ICD excluded, unless noted)
Freeman, 2012 22095828	356,515	82%	04/06-03/10	1473	Epicardial lead placement Missing physician data
Haines, 2011 21537001	268,701	78%	01/06-06/08	1300	Pts requiring thoracotomy Includes patients with prior ICD
Cheng, 2010 21050975	226,764	nd	04/06-09/08	nd	
Freeman, 2010 20863954	224,233	81%	01/06-12/08	1356	Epicardial lead placement Hospitals not reporting all implants per quarter of data
Aggarwal, 2009 19879533	164,069	68%†	01/06-12/07	1241	Missing ESRD status data
Peterson, 2009 19221223	161,470	72%	01/06-12/07	1224	
Tsai, 2011 21878667	150,264	100%	01/06-12/08	nd	Secondary prevention Hospitals only submitting data on Medicare patients
Curtis, 2009 19383957	111,293	83%	01/06-06/07	1062	Age <18 Epicardial lead placement Physician <10 procedures during study
Dewland, 2011 21867834	104,049	82%	01/06-12/07	nd	Biventricular ICD
Wei, 2011 21487093	53,198	77%†	01/06-12/08	1300	No data for serum BNP May include prior ICD as this is not stated as exclusion
Tsai, 2011 21883101 Subgroup only	44,805	100%	01/06-12/08	nd	Do not meet MADIT II criteria, which are MI >40 days, LVEF ≤ 30%, NYHA I, II or III

ESRD=end stage renal disease; ICD=implantable cardioverter–defibrillator; LVEF=left ventricular ejection fraction; MADIT II=Multicenter Automatic Defibrillator Implantation Trial II; MI=myocardial infarction; NCDR=National Cardiovascular Data Registry; nd=not documented; NYHA=New York Heart Association; PMID=PubMed ID

* Number of sites is limited to sites achieving NCDR Data Reporting Quality thresholds. It is unclear if and why this would be different in studies with same time period.
† Calculated

Appendix Table 13. Percentage of patients with early (in-hospital) adverse events in NCDR ICD database

Outcomes	Range*	Freeman 2012 22095828 356,515	Haines 2011 21537001 268,701	Cheng 2010 21050975 226,764	Freeman 2010 20863954 224,233	Aggarwal 2009 19879533 164,069	Peterson 2009 19221223 161,470	Tsai 2011 21878667 150,264	Curtis 2009 19383957 111,293	Dewland 2011 21867834 104,049	Wei 2011* 21487093 53,198
Any adverse event	2.77–3.55	3.08	3.05	--	3.19	3.6†	3.55	3.26	3.7	2.77†	4.59†
Any serious adverse event	1.17–1.35	1.17	--	--	1.20	1.3†	1.35	1.2†‡	--	--	--
Any adverse event or death	1.5–3.37	--	3.2	--	--	--	--	3.37	1.5	--	1.97†
Arteriovenous fistula	<0.1	--	<0.01	--	--	0.01†	0.01	0	<0.1	<0.01†	0.01†
Cardiac arrest	0.26–0.34	0.29	0.30	0.32†	0.3	0.3†	0.34	0.26	0.3	0.28†	0.69†
Cardiac perforation	0.06–0.1	--	0.07	0.08†	--	0.08†	0.08	0.07	0.1	0.06†	0.07†
Cardiac valve injury	<0.1	--	<0.01	--	--	§	0	--	<0.1	<0.01†	--
Conduction block	0.03–0.1	--	0.03	--	--	0.04†	0.04	0.04	0.1	0.03†	0.04†
Coronary venous dissection	0.08–0.15	0.12	0.12	--	--	0.15†	0.15	--	0.1	0.08†	0.19†
Drug reaction	0.09–0.11	--	0.09	0.09†	--	0.1†	0.11	--	0.1	0.10†	0.15†
Hematoma	0.84–1.1	0.86	0.93	1.01†	--	1.0†	1.06	0.94	1.1	0.84†	1.39†
Hemothorax	0.07–0.1	--	0.08	0.09†	0.9	0.1†	0.10	0.09	0.1	0.07†	0.12†
Infection related to device	<0.1	--	0.03	0.02†	--	0.03†	0.03	--	<0.1	0.03*	0.06*
Lead dislodgement	0.73–1.2	1.02	0.93	1.2	1.0	1.1†	1.09	--	1.0	0.73†	1.24†
Myocardial infarction	<0.1	--	0.02	--	--	0.03†	0.03	0.03	<0.1	0.03†	0.05†
Pericardial tamponade	0.07–0.1	--	0.07	--	--	0.1†	0.09	0.10	0.1	0.07†	0.08†
Peripheral embolism	<0.1	--	0.03	0.03†	--	0.03†	0.03	--	0	0.03†	0.06†
Peripheral nerve injury	<0.1	--	<0.01	--	--	§	0	--	<0.1	<0.01†	0.01†
Phlebitis, deep	<0.1	--	0.02	--	--	0.03†	0.03	--	<0.1	0.02†	0.06†
Phlebitis, superficial	0.04–0.1	--	0.04	0.04†	--	0.1†	0.05	--	0.1	0.05†	0.07†
Pneumothorax	0.42–0.51	0.44	0.42	0.48†	0.5	0.5†	0.51	0.45	0.5	0.46†	0.58†
Stroke/CVA	0.05–0.1	--	0.06	--	--	0.1†	0.07	0.05	0.1	0.06†	0.12†
Transient ischemic attack	<0.1	--	0.02	--	--	0.02†	0.02	0.03	<0.1	0.02†	0.04†

CVA=cerebrovascular accident; ICD=implantable cardioverter–defibrillator; NCDR=National Cardiovascular Data Registry; PMID=PubMed ID

* Data from Wei, 2011 PMID 21487093 are outliers and are not included. All patients in this study had B-type natriuretic peptide (BNP) measurement which may represent patients with heart failure. Also the study did not explicitly exclude patients with prior ICD.
† Calculated.
‡ From figure.
§ Likely error in original paper: rate for cardiac valve injury (3%) and peripheral nerve injury (8%) are inconsistent with other studies from NCDR ICD database.

Appendix Table 14: P values for comparisons of early (in-hospital) adverse events by patient subgroup in the NCDR ICD database

	Primary vs. Secondary Prevention	Dual- vs. Single-chamber ICD*	CRT-D vs. Single-chamber ICD*	Older age†	Female‡	Race / Ethnicity	DM	ESRD§	Lower physician implant volume‖	Lower hospital implant volume¶
Any adverse event	--	P<0.001 (I) P<0.05** (B) nd (A,D,H)	P<0.05** (B) nd (A,D,H)	P<0.001 (K) P<0.05**(B)†† nd (G)	P<0.001 (F) P<0.05** (B)	--	--	P<0.0001 (E)	P<0.0001 (A)	P<0.0001 (D) nd (A)
Any serious adverse event	--	nd (A,D)	nd (A,D)	nd (G)	P<0.001 (F)	--	--	P<0.0001 (E)	P<0.0001 (A)	P<0.0001 (D)
Any adverse event or death	NS (B)	P<0.001 (G) nd (H)	P<0.001 (G) nd (H)	P<0.0001 (B) P<0.05 (G)‡‡	P<0.0001 (B) P<0.001(G)	P<0.01 (G)§§ Higher for Black	NS (B)	P<0.0001 (B) P<0.001 (G)	--	--
Arteriovenous fistula	--	NS (I) ¶¶	--	nd (G) ¶¶	NS (F) ¶¶	--	--	NS (E)	--	--
Cardiac arrest	--	P=0.01 (I) nd (A)	nd (A)	nd (G)	NS (F)	--	--	P<0.0001 (E)	--	--
Cardiac perforation	--	NS (I)	--	nd (G) ¶¶	P<0.001 (F)	--	--	NS (E)	--	--
Cardiac valve injury	--	NS (I) ¶¶	--	--	NS (F) ¶¶	--	--	***	--	--
Conduction block	--	NS (I) ¶¶	--	nd (G) ¶¶	P<0.001 (F)	--	--	NS (E)	--	--
Coronary venous dissection	--	P<0.001 (I) ¶¶ nd (A)	nd (A)	--	P<0.001 (F)	--	--	P=0.05 (E) § Lower in ESRD	--	--
Drug reaction	--	NS (I)	--	--	P=0.015 (F)	--	--	P<0.0001 (E)	--	--
Hemothorax	--	NS (I)	--	nd (G)	P<0.001 (F)	--	--	P=0.01 (E)	--	--
Hematoma	--	P<0.001 (I) nd (A)	nd (A)	nd (G)	NS (F)	--	--	P<0.0001 (E)	--	--
Infection related to device	--	NS (I)	--	--	NS (F)	--	--	NS (E)	--	--
Lead dislodgement	--	P<0.001 (I) P<0.05** (C) nd (A)	P<0.05(C) ¶¶ nd (A)	NS (C)	P=0.002 (F) P<0.001 (C)	P=0.005 (C) Higher for White†††	NS (C)	NS (E)	--	--
Myocardial infarction	--	P=0.05 (I) ¶¶	--	nd (G) ¶¶	NS (F)	--	--	NS (E)	--	--
Pericardial tamponade	--	P=0.01 (I)	--	nd (G)	P<0.001 (F)	--	--	NS (E)	--	--
Peripheral nerve injury	--	NS (I) ¶¶	--	--	NS (F) ¶¶	--	--	***	--	--

	Primary vs. Secondary Prevention	Dual- vs. Single-chamber ICD*	CRT-D vs. Single-chamber ICD*	Older age†	Female‡	Race / Ethnicity	DM	ESRD§	Lower physician implant volume‖	Lower hospital implant volume¶
Peripheral embolism	--	NS (I) ¶¶	--	--	P=0.014 (F)	--	--	NS (E)	--	--
Phlebitis - deep	--	NS (I) ¶¶	--	--	P=0.008 (F)	--	--	NS (E)	--	--
Phlebitis - superficial	--	P=0.009(I)	--	--	NS (F)	--	--	NS (E)	--	--
Pneumothorax	--	P<0.001 (I) nd (A)	nd (A)	nd (G)	P<0.001 (F)	--	--	NS (E)	--	--
Stroke/CVA	--	NS (I)	--	nd (G) ¶¶	NS (F)	--	--	NS (E)	--	--
Transient ischemic attack	--	NS (I) ¶¶	--	nd (G) ¶¶	NS (F) ¶¶	--	--	NS (E)	--	--
Number of papers (reporting statistics)	1 (1)	7 (4)	5 (2)	4 (3)	4 (4)	2 (2)	2 (2)	4 (4)	1 (1)	2 (1)

A-J in parentheses indicate the specific studies. See Study Key, below.

P values <0.05 indicate statistically higher rates of AE in subgroup in column header, unless otherwise noted. NS indicates no statistical difference in AE between subgroups. "nd" indicates paper reported rates of AE by subgroup but did not report statistical comparison between groups.

AE=adverse event; CRT-D=cardiac resynchronization therapy-defibrillator; CVA=cerebrovascular accident; DM=diabetes mellitus; ESRD=end-stage renal disease; ICD=implantable cardioverter-defibrillator; NCDR=National Cardiovascular Data Registry;

*   More leads resulted in higher rates of adverse events unless difference between groups.
†   Adverse events were higher in older patients unless difference between groups NS. Age cutoffs varied between papers.
‡   Female sex resulted in higher rates of adverse events, unless difference between groups NS.
§   Rate of adverse events are higher in patients with ESRD unless difference between groups NS, with the following exception: rates of coronary venous dissection are 0.06% and 0.15%, for ESRD and non-ESRD groups, respectively (E).
‖   Rates of adverse events decrease with higher physician implant volume, p=p trend.
¶   Rates of adverse events decrease with higher hospital implant volume, p=p trend.
**   Paper reports odds or hazards ratio with confidence interval that does not cross 1.0. No p-value reported.
††   Rates of any adverse event increased statistically across the age groups ≤65, 65-75 and ≥75 (K) and with age >70 (B).
‡‡   Rates of any adverse event or death were statistically for age ≥75 (G) and with age >70 (B).
§§   Rates of any adverse event or death are higher in black subgroup, reference group not documented (G).
¶¶   Less than 10 events in at least one subgroup.
***   Paper reports NS between groups. However rate data is inconsistent in order of magnitude within paper and with other papers.
†††   Rates of lead dislodgement differed across White, Black, Hispanic and Other subgroups with Whites having more events (C).

C-30

Study Key (author, year, PubMed ID)

A	Freeman, 2012	22095828	E	Aggarwal, 2009	19879533	I	Dewland, 2011	21867834
B	Haines, 2011	21537001	F	Peterson, 2009	19221223	J	Wei, 2011	21487093
C	Cheng, 2010	21050975	G	Tsai, 2011	21878667	K	Tsai, 2011	21883101
D	Freeman, 2010	20863954	H	Curtis, 2009	19383957			

Appendix Table 15. Study characteristics of comparative studies of ICDs with adverse event data

Study Author, Year PMID	Country	N	Primary Prevention	Study Duration	No. Sites	Study Design	Inclusion/Exclusion Criteria	Age (Mean)	Male (%)
ICD vs. CRT-D									
ALTITUDE Saxon, 2010 21098452	US	185,778	nd	2006-05/09*	2096	Prospective cohort	Inclusion: All patients receiving ICD or CRT-D with Boston Scientific remote monitoring device	67	74%
MADIT-CRT Moss , 2009, 19723701	US	1,820	100%	12/04-04/08	110	RCT	Inclusion: Age ≥21, ischemic cardiomyopathy (NYHA class I or II) or nonischemic cardiomyopathy (NYHA class II only), sinus rhythm, ejection fraction ≤30% and prolonged intraventricular conduction with a QRS duration ≥130 msec Exclusion: An existing indication for CRT, implanted pacemaker, ICD or CRT, NYHA class III or IV symptopms, previous CABG, percutaneous coronary intervention, or MI within 3 mo; atrial fibrillation within 1 mo	65	75%
RAFT Tang, 2010 21073365 Parkash, 2012 23159551	Canada, Europe, Turkey, Australia	1798	86%	01/03-08/10	34	RCT	Inclusion: Primary or secondary prevention, NHYA class II or III symptoms of heart failure despite receiving optimal medical therapy, LVEF ≤30%, ischemic or nonischemic causes, an intrinsic QRS duration ≥120 msec or paced QRS duration ≥200 msec, sinus rhythm or permanent atrial fibrillation or flutter with a controlled ventricular rate or planned atrioventricular-junction ablation after device implantation. Exclusion: Major coexisting illness or a recent cardiovascular event.	66	83%
MENDMI Chung, 2010 20852059	US	80	100%	04/05-03/08	nd	RCT	Inclusion: Recent MI, QRS duration <120 msec, LVEF ≤35%, abnormal wall motion in at least 5 of 16 possible segments measured 2 to 14 days after presentation Exclusion: Permanent or persistent atrial tachyarrhythmia, cardiogenic shock, 2° or 3° heart block, marked renal dysfunction, CABG within 30 days, NYHA class IV, previous ICD or pacemaker or CRT device.	57	75%

Study Author, Year PMID	Country	N	Primary Prevention	Study Duration	No. Sites	Study Design	Inclusion/Exclusion Criteria	Age (Mean)	Male (%)
Single- vs. Dual- Chamber									
ADRIA Sticherling, 2011 21156772	Germany & Switzerland	249	nd	nd	10	RCT	Inclusion: age≥18, indication for ICD; Exclusion: Antibradycardia pacing, permanent atrial fibrillation	63	87%

ADRIA= A+ versus DR Clinical Investigation of Arrhythmia Discrimination; ALTITUDE= the acronym is undefined CABG=Coronary Artery Bypass Graft; CRT-D=cardiac resynchronization therapy-defibrillator; ICD=implantable cardioverter–defibrillator; LVEF=left ventricular ejection fraction; MADIT-CRT=Multicenter Automatic Defibrillator Implantation Trial with Cardiac Resynchronization Therapy; MENDMI=Prevention of Myocardial Enlargement and Dilation Post Myocardial Infarction Study; MI=myocardial infarction; nd=not documented; No=number; NYHA=New York Heart Association; PMID=PubMed ID; RAFT= Resynchronization–Defibrillation for Ambulatory Heart Failure Trial; RCT=randomized, controlled trial; US=Unitec States

*Month in 2006 in which data collection began was not documented.

Appendix Table 16. Adverse events from comparative studies of ICDs

Study Author, Year PMID	N	Primary Prevention	Intervention	Early Adverse Events			Late Adverse Events & Inappropriate shock		
				Followup	Outcome	% (P value*)	Followup	Outcome	% (P value*)
ICD vs. CRT-D									
ALTITUDE Saxon, 2010 21098452	185,778	nd	ICD vs. CRT-D		--		5 y	Inappropriate shocks	16% vs. 17%
MADIT-CRT Moss, 2009 19723701	1,820	100%	ICD vs. CRT-D	In-hospital	Coronary venous dissection with pericardial effusion	0% vs. 0.5%	2.4 y	Total device-related AE	5.2 vs. 4.5 †
				30 days	Pneumothorax	0.8% vs. 1.7%			
					Infection	0.70% vs. 1.10%			
					Pocket hematoma req. evacuation	2.5% vs. 3.3%			
RAFT Tang, 2010 21073365	1798	86%	ICD vs. CRT-D	30 days	Hemothorax or pneumothorax	0.9% vs. 1.2%		--	
					Hematoma req. intervention	1.2% vs.1.6%			
					Pocket infection req. intervention	1.8% vs. 2.4%			
					Lead dislodgement req. intervention	2.2% vs. 6.9%			
					Pocket problems req. revision	0.1% vs. 0.5%			
					Coronary sinus dissection	0% vs. 1.2%			
MENDMI Chung, 2010 20852059	80	100%	ICD vs. CRT-D		--		1 y	Total AE	42% vs. 52% (NS) ‡
Single- vs. Dual- Chamber									
ADRIA Sticherling, 2011 21156772	249	nd	Single-chamber vs. dual-chamber ICD §	In-hospital	Pneumothorax	0.8% vs. 0.8% (NS)‖	1 y	Inappropriate shocks	5.6% vs. 5.6%¶
					Ventricular perforation	0% vs. 0.8% (NS)‖		Ventricular lead-related AE	5.6% vs. 4.0% (NS)**

ADRIA= A+ versus DR Clinical Investigation of Arrhythmia Discrimination; AE=adverse events; ALTITUDE= the acronym is undefined; CRT-D=cardiac resynchronization therapy-defibrillator; ICD=implantable cardioverter–defibrillator; MADIT-CRT=Multicenter Automatic Defibrillator Implantation Trial with Cardiac Resynchronization Therapy; MENDMI=Prevention of Myocardial Enlargement and Dilation Post Myocardial Infarction Study; nd=not documented; PMID=PubMed ID; req=requiring; y=year

* P-value provided only if documented.
† Total device-related AE per 100 device-months
‡ Data calculated. Prespecified composite AE: Left ventricular lead dislodgement, postimplantation left ventricular lead repositioning, permanent failure to deliver biventricular pacing, ventricular tachyarrythmia, hospitalization due to cardiac causes and all-cause mortality.
§ ICD with a single-lead with an integrated atrial sensing rings mounted 15 to 18 cm from the tip of the ICD lead versus a dual lead (dual chamber) ICD
‖ Data calculated

¶ Data calculated. 34 episodes in 7 patients vs. 12 episodes in 7 patients.
** Data calculated. Ventricular lead dislocation or high threshold. Follow-up time unclear (in-hospital or 12 months)

Appendix Table 17. Characteristics of studies of late adverse events and inappropriate shock

Author, Year PMID, Country	N	Primary Prevention	Study Duration	# Sites	Study Design	Inclusion/Exclusion Criteria	Age (mean)	Male (%)
ICD arms from RCTs*								
SCD-HeFT Bardy, 2005 15659722, US	829	100%	09/97-10/03	multiple	RCT	Inclusion: Age≥18, NYHA II-III, CHF due to ischemic or nonischemic causes, LVEF ≤35%	60 median	77[†]
MADIT II Moss, 2002 11907286 US & Europe	742	100%	07/97-11/01	76	RCT	Inclusion: Age ≥21, >1 mo since MI and LVEF≤30 within 3 mo before entry, primary prevention Exclusion: Coronary revascularization within 3 mo, MI within 1 mo, NYHA class IV, advanced cerebrovascular disease	64	84
Other Studies								
Birnie, 2012 22311781, Canada	3,169	67%	12/03-11/07	11	Retrospective cohort	Inclusion: All pts receiving ICDs with Sprint Fidelis leads	63	82[†]
Bode, 2012 22753865, Germany	903	nd	01/93-12/09 (implant date)	1	Retrospective cohort	Inclusion: All pts receiving first transvenous ICD	64	81
Borleffs, 2009 19808497, NL	2,068[‡]	55%	1992-02/08	1	Prospective cohort	Inclusion: All pts receiving ICDs Exclusion: Receiving abdominal system or leads with coaxial construction or polyurethane coating	61	80
Brumberg, 2012 22519559, US	621	nd	05/04-12/07 (implant date)	1	Retrospective cohort	Inclusion: All pts receiving initial ICD, revision or upgrade with Fidelis lead	66	75
Brullman, 2012 22154315 Austria, Switzerland	936§	42%[†]	1987-2009 (implant dates)	2	Prospective cohort	Inclusion: Age ≥18 receiving first ICD for primary or secondary prevention or syncope [2]	63 median	85
Charytan, 2011 21664735, US	9,528	<50%	1994-2006	nd	Registry	Inclusion: Age ≥21, all dialysis pts in USRDS implanted with ICD or CRT	65	70
Cheung, 2012 22923271, US	732	91%	09/04-10/07 (implant date)	1	Retrospective cohort	Inclusion: All pts receiving Sprint Fidelis leads Exclusion: <90 days followup	67	76[†]
De Bie, 2012 22056722, NL	2,476[‡]	66%	01/00-09/09 (implant date)	1	Prospective cohort	Inclusion: All pts receiving first ICD or CRT-D	62	79
Desai, 2010 20403488, US	549	nd	nd	1	Retrospective cohort	Inclusion: Pts with heart failure receiving ICDs	74	79[†]
Dichtl, 2011 21678454 Austria, Switzerland	1,117§	40%	nd	2	Prospective cohort	nd	nd [∥]	81
RIGHT, Gold, 2012 21978966 US, Canada, Europe	1962	85%[†]	nd	130	RCT	Inclusion: Pts scheduled to receive ICD	64	79[†]

Author, Year PMID, Country	N	Primary Prevention	Study Duration	# Sites	Study Design	Inclusion/Exclusion Criteria	Age (mean)	Male (%)
Gradaus, 2003 12914630 Germany	3,344	7.1%	01/98-10/00 (implant date)	62	Retrospective cohort	Inclusion: All pts receiving ICDs	61	80
Hauser, 2002 22396584, US	2,710	75%†	11/01-11/09	3	Retrospective cohort	Inclusion: All pts receiving Sprint Fidelis or Quattro Secure leads	64†	77†
Kleeman, 2012 22313314, Germany	1,411	32%†	1992-05/08 (implant date)	1	Prospective cohort	Inclusion: pts receiving ICDs for primary or secondary prevention	66	79†
Landolina, 2011 21576653 Italy	3,253	87%	2004-2009 (implant date)	117	Prospective cohort	Inclusion: Consecutive pts receiving first single- or dual-chamber ICD or CRT-D systems including pts with preexisting pacemakers.	67	80
Larsen, 2010 20186244 New Zealand	702	27%†	01/00-12/07 (implant date)	2	Retrospective cohort	Inclusion: All pts receiving first ICD	53	77
Lee, 2010 20170816 Canada	3,340¶	70%†	02/07-05/09	nd	Registry	Inclusion: De novo single- or dual-chamber ICD or CRT-D. Exclusion: <45 day followup	64	79
Lyman, 2011 21795298, US	38,992	100	1997-2006	nd	Retrospective cohort	Inclusion: All primary ICD implantation admissions	66	77
MacFadden, 2012 22312139, Canada	5,213¶	72%†	02/07-07/10	nd	Registry	Inclusion: De novo single- or dual-chamber ICD or CRT-D for primary or secondary prevention	65	79
Morrison, 2011 21737019, US	2,671	75%	11/01-12/08 (implant date)	3	Prospective cohort	Inclusion: All pts receiving ICDs with Sprint Fidelis or Quattro Secure leads	65†	77†
MADIT-RIT Moss, 2012 23131066 US & other**	1,500	100%	09/09-07/12	98	RCT	Inclusion: ≥21 yrs, ischemic or nonischemic heart disease, sinus rhythm, standard indication for ICD or CRT-D for primary prevention Exclusion: Prior ICD, Pacemaker or CRT; Atrial fibrillation; CABG, PCI or MI within 3 mo	63†	71†
RAFT Parkash, 2012 23159551	1787	86%	01/03-08/10	34	RCT	Inclusion: Primary or secondary prevention, NHYA class II or III, LVEF ≤30%, ischemic or nonischemic causes, an intrinsic QRS duration ≥120 msec or paced QRS duration ≥200 msec. (See Appendix Table 14) Exclusion: Major coexisting illness or a recent cardiovascular event.	66	83
Porterfield, 2010 19925609 US, Germany	15,387	nd	06/01-11/07	28	Retrospective cohort	Inclusion: Pts implanted with Riata lead model numbers from 1500 and 7000 series	66	76
Remmelts, 2009 19325900, NL	667	nd	01/96-10/06 (implant date)	1	Retrospective cohort	Inclusion: All pts receiving first ICD Exclusion: Pulse generator inserted in abdominal	58	77

Author, Year PMID, Country	N	Primary Prevention	Study Duration	# Sites	Study Design	Inclusion/Exclusion Criteria	Age (mean)	Male (%)
INTRINSIC RV Sandesara, 2011 21086086, US	1,528	nd	nd	108	Post-hoc analysis of RCT	Inclusion: Indication for ICD and VITALITY AVT ICD implanted pocket or epicardial lead system	65	81†
ALTITUDE Saxon, 2010 21098452, US	185,778	nd	2006-05/09	2096	Prospective cohort	Inclusion: All pts receiving ICD or CRT-D with Boston Scientific remote monitoring device	68†	75†
Schaer, 2011 21712284, NL	536	100%	1998-2008	2	Retrospective cohort	Inclusion: All pts with CAD receiving ICD or CRT-D for primary prevention	63	88
Sengupta, 2012 22314669 US	1644	55%	08/94-05/04 (implant date)	1	Retrospective cohort	Inclusion: All pts receiving first ICD Exclusion: Pts receiving investigational ICDs or ICDs with unclear advisory/non-advisory status	63	78
Sweeney,2012 22387371, US Subgroups only	1,464	100%	08/05-04/11	134	Prospective cohort	Inclusion:All pts receiving Medtronic ICD or CRT-D for primary prevention and LVEF ≤35%	67	72
Sweeney, 2010 20185109, US	2,135	67%	nd	nd	Post-hoc analysis of 4 Trials††	Inclusion:All pts had Medtronic ICDs implanted less than 4 wks before enrollment	66	80
PainFree RX II Sweeney, 2005 15927965, US Subgroups only	582‡‡	43%†	nd	nd	RCT	Inclusion: Pts receiving ICDs Exclusion: Pts unlikely to have substrate for stable monomorphic VT susceptible to pace termination	68	79
Thijssen,2012 22094073, NL	3,194‡	62%	1996-04/11	1	Prospective cohort	Inclusion: All pts receiving ICDs	62	78
Tsai, 2010 19262366, US	1,060	nd	nd	1	Retrospective cohort	Inclusion: All pts receiving ICDs	70	80
Tzogias, 2012 22314669, US	971	85%	09/04-07/07 (implant date)	1	Retrospective cohort	Inclusion: Al pts receiving Sprint Fidelis 6949 lead	68	73
Van Rees, 2012 22352338, NL	1,602‡	58%	1996-02/11	1	Prospective cohort	Inclusion: All pts receiving ICDs with transvenous leads Exclusion: Pts with Sprint Fidelis or Riata leads	61	80
Van Rees, 2011 21272746, NL Subgroups only	1,544‡	56%	1996-2006	1	Prospective cohort	Inclusion: All pts receiving ICDs	61	79
Van Rees, 2012 21920909, NL Subgroups only	1,395‡	100%	01/96-01/09	1	Prospective cohort	Inclusion: All pts receiving ICDs for primary prevention Exclusion: Congenital structural or monogenetic heart disease	63	79
Van Welsenes 2011 21208947, NL	2,134‡	61%	1996-01/08	1	Prospective cohort	Inclusion: All pts receiving ICD Exclusion: Congenital monogenetic cardiac	63	81†

Author, Year PMID, Country	N	Primary Prevention	Study Duration	# Sites	Study Design	Inclusion/Exclusion Criteria	Age (mean)	Male (%)
						disease, hypertrophic obstructive cardiomyopathy, long-QT syndrome, Brugada syndrome, and idiopathic VF, related to an increased risk of cardiac arrhythmia		
TRUST Varma, 2010 20716717, US	1,339	73%[†]	08/05–05/09	102	RCT (remote monitoring vs. conventional)	Inclusion: Recipients of single- or dual-chamber ICDs for class I/II indications Exclusion: Pacemaker dependent	64[†]	72[†]

ALTITUDE=acronym is undefined; CABG=coronary artery bypass grafting; CAD=coronary artery disease; CHF=congestive heart failure; CRT-D=cardiac resynchronization therapy-defibrillator; ICD=implantable cardioverter–defibrillator; INTRINSIC RV= Inhibition of Unnecessary RV Pacing with AV Search Hysteresis in ICDs; LV=F=left ventricular ejection fraction; MADIT II= Multicenter Automatic Defibrillator Implantation Trial II; MADIT-RIT= Multicenter automatic defibrillator implantation trial: reduce inappropriate therapy; MI=myocardial infarction; mo=month; nd=not documented; NL: Netherlands; NYHA=New York Heart Association; PCI=percutaneous coronary intervention; PMID:=PubMed ID; pts=patients; RCT=randomized, controlled trial; RIGHT=Rhythm ID Goes Head to Head Trial; RV=right ventricular; SCD-HeFT= Sudden Cardiac Death in Heart Failure Trial; TRUST= Lumos-T Safely Reduces Routine Office Device Follow Up; US=United States; USRDS=United States Renal Data System; VF=ventricular fibrillation; VT=ventricular tachycardia

* Includes ICD arm of trials from Key Question 1 with ≥500 patients with ICDs and nonICD control groups.

† calculated

‡ Likely patient overlap between Van Welsenes [21208947], Borleffs [19808497], de Bie [22056722], Thijssen [22094073], Van Rees [21920909], [22352338] and [21272746]. All data from Leiden University Medical Center Cardiology Information System (EPD-Vision).

§ Likely patient overlap between Brullmar [22154315] and Ditchl [21678454].

|| 19.3% of patients age >70yr

¶ Patients in Lee [20170816] included in MacFadden [22312139].

** US, Canada, Israel, Japan and Europe

†† Four trials incorporating ATP to reduce shocks (PainFREE Rx, PainFREE Rx II, EMPIRIC, and PREPARE)

‡‡ All patients included in Sweeney, 2010, PMID 20185109

Appendix Table 18. Inappropriate shock (among studies with N ≥500)

Study Author, Year PMID	N	Mean followup	Device Type	Model	Patients with Inappropriate Shock (%)	Between Arm Comparison
Comparative studies						
Morrison, 2011 21737019	1,030 / 1,641	34 mo / 40 mo	ICD or CRT-D	Medtronic Sprint Fidelis 6931, 6948, 6949 / Medtronic Quattro Secure 6947	20% / 14%	P<0.001
RIGHT Gold, 2012 21978966	985 / 977	18 mo	Single- or dual-chamber ICD	Guidant Vitality 2 with Rhythm ID / Medtronic Maximo Marquis, Intrinsic, Virtuoso, or Entrust with Wavelet or Enhanced PR logic	18%* / 12%*	P<0.001†
MADIT-RIT Moss, 2012 23131066	514 / 500 / 486	17 mo*	Dual-chamber ICD or CRT-D	Conventional programming‡ / High-rate therapy‡ / Delayed therapy‡	6% / 3% / 3%	-- / P=0.01 vs. conventional / P=0.03 vs. conventional
ICD arms from RCTs[b]						
SCD-HeFT Bardy, 2005 15659722	829	46 mo median	Single-chamber ICD	Medtronic 7223	2.4% per year	--
Other Studies						
ALTITUDE[||] Saxon, 2010 21098452	185,778	60 mo	Single- or dual-chamber ICD or CRT-D	Boston Scientific remote-monitoring capable device	16%*[||]	--
Brullman, 2012 22154315	936[¶]	43 mo	Single- or dual-chamber ICD or CRT-D	nd	21%	--
Van Welsenes, 2011 21208947	2,134	41 mo*	Single- or dual-chamber ICD or CRT-D	Biotronik, Medtronic, Boston Scientific/ Guidant, St. Jude Medical/Ventritex	14%**	--
Desai, 2010 20403488	549	41 mo[††]	ICD	nd	13%‡‡	--
Larsen, 2010 20186244	702	40 mo median	Single- or dual-chamber ICD or CRT-D	nd	16%	--
Kleemann, 2012 22313314	1,411	36 mo*	Single- or dual-chamber ICD or CRT-D	Biotronik, Medtronic, ELA Medical, Guidant, St. Jude Medical	21%[§§]	--
Dichtl, 2011 21678454	1,117[¶]	35 mo*	Single- or dual-chamber ICD or CRT-D	nd	21%	--
Schaer, 2011 21712284	536	30 mo	Single- or dual-chamber ICD or CRT-D	nd	8.0%	--
MacFadden, 2012 22312139	5,213	12 mo	Single- or dual-chamber ICD or CRT-D	nd	3.0%	--
INTRINSIC RV Sandesara,2011 21086086	1,528	12 mo	Dual-chamber ICD	Guidant Vitality AVT	6.3%*	

Study Author, Year PMID	N	Mean followup	Device Type	Model	Patients with Inappropriate Shock (%)	Between Arm Comparison
Sweeney, 2010 20185109	2,135	12 mo*	ICD	Medtronic	8.6%*‖‖‖	

ATP=antitachycardia pacing; bpm=beats per minute; CRT-D=cardiac resynchronization therapy-defibrillator; ICD=implantable cardioverter–defibrillator; mo=month; nd=not documented; PMID=PubMed ID; VF=ventricular fibrillation; VT=ventricular tachycardia. For study name acronyms see Appendix Table 16.

*   calculated

†   Single chamber ICDs Guidant vs. Medtronic p=0.003; dual chamber ICDs Guidant vs. Medtronic p=0.006

‡   Boston Scientific ICDs. Conventional programming: For 170 bpm (VT), 2.5 second delay, atrial discriminators on, ATP+shock. For 200 bpm (VF) 1.0 second delay, ATP+shock. High rate therapy: For 170 bpm (VT), monitor only. For 200 bpm (VF) 2.5 second delay, ATP+shock Delayed therapy For 170 bpm (VT-1), rhythm detection on, 60 second delay, ATP+shock For 200 bpm (VT) rhythm detection on, 12 second delay ATP+shock. For 250 bpm (VF) 2.5 second delay ATP+shock. In all devices, ATP was followed by shock therapy only if pacing did not terminate the tachycardia.

§   Includes ICD arm of trials from Key Question 1 with ≥500 patients with ICDs and nonICD control groups.

‖   ALTITUDE study is also included in Appendix Table 15

¶   Likely patient overlap between Brullman [22154315] and Ditchl [21678454].

**   Patients receiving inappropriate shocks experienced 2.9 +/- 4.5 shocks (mean.) Additional papers published from EPD-Vision Database with smaller numbers of patients and similar or shorter follow-up periods report rates of inappropriate shocks ranging from 10%-15% [PMID 21272746, 20185038, 20639206].

††   Unclear if follow-up begins at implantation.

‡‡   187 inappropriate shocks in 71 patients

§§   297 patients received 948 inappropriate shocks

‖‖‖   Four trials incorporating ATP to reduce shocks (PainFREE Rx, PainFREE Rx II, EMPIRIC, and PREPARE). Pain FREE RX II trial alone reports 9.1% of patients experiencing inappropriate shocks (PMID 15927965) with a followup of 11 months.

Appendix Table 19. Late adverse events: Device- and lead-related adverse events

Study Author, Year PMID	N	Mean Followup	Device Type [Model]*	Device-Related Adverse Events	%	/100 Pt-Y	Lead-Related Adverse Events	%	/100 Pt-Y
ICD arms from RCTs†									
MADIT II Moss, 2002 11907286	742	20 mo	ICD [Guidant]	--			Lead problems requiring surgical intervention	1.8%	--
Other Studies									
Hauser, 2002 22396584	1,675	86 mo maximum	ICD [Quattro Secure 6947]	--			Lead failure	1.4%	--
Sengupta, 2012 22314669	940	70 mo	Single- or dual-chamber ICD or CRT-D	Device malfunction (P<0.001 vs. advisory)	1.6%	--			
Thijssen, 2012 22094073	3,194‡	49 mo	Single- or dual-chamber ICD or CRT-D [Multiple] §	System malfunction requiring replacement	2.6%	--			
Bode, 2012 22753865	903	49 mo	ICD [High voltage RV lead]	--			High voltage lead defect	7.0%	--
Brullman, 2012 22154315	936‖	43 mo	Single- or dual-chamber ICD or CRT-D	--			Lead revision	19%	--
van Rees, 2012 22352338	1,602‡	41 mo	ICD¶	--			Lead failure	3.9%	1.14
							Cumulative lead failure at 8 yr	11.5%	--
Morrison, 2011 21737019	1,641	40 mo	ICD or CRT-D [Quattro Secure 6947]	--			Lead survival: 98.7%	--	--
RAFT Parkash, 2012 23159551	969	39 mo median	ICD or CRT-D	--			Lead failure	0.2%	--
Tsai, 2010 19262366	1,060	38 mo	ICD	ICD malfunction requiring replacement	0.5%	--	Lead repositioning required	0.3%	--
							Lead fracture requiring revision	3.4%	
Borleffs, 2009 19808497	2,068‡	36 mo	Single- or dual-chamber ICD or CRT-D [Multiple] §	--			Lead failure	3.8%	1.4**
							Lead dislodgement within 6 mo	0.6%††	--
Dichtl, 2011 21678454	1,117‖	35 mo††	Single- or dual-chamber ICD or CRT-D	--			Lead dysfunction (undefined)	16.5%	--
Porterfield, 2010 19925609	15,387	18.0 mo	ICD or CRT-D [St. Jude Riata leads 1500 or 7000 series]	--			Total lead-related AE‡‡	3.6%§§	--
							Lead dislodgement	0.9%	--
							Lead malfunction, electrical ‖‖	0.5%	--
							Lead malfunction, other¶¶	1.9%	--

Study Author, Year PMID	N	Mean Followup	Device Type [Model]*	Device-Related Adverse Events	%	/100 Pt-Y	Lead-Related Adverse Events	%	/100 Pt-Y
Landolina, 2011 21576653	3,253	18 mo median	Single- or dual-chamber ICD or CRT-D [Medtronic]	ICD surgical revision	6.4%††	5.2***	Lead malfunction	--	1.2†††
							Lead dislodgement	--	2.8†††
Charytan, 2011 21664735	9,528 ESRD	16.8 mo††	ICD or CRT-D	Generator replacement	--	3.9	Lead removal / change	--	3.4
TRUST Varma, 2010 20716717	1,339	13.4 mo††	Single- or dual-chamber ICD [Biotronik] ‡‡	ICD replacement	<0.1%††	0.1	Lead revision	0.9%††	0.8
							Lead replacement	0.4%††	0.34
							ICD explanted due to lead fracture	<0.1%	0.07
Lyman, 2011 21795298	38,992	3 mo 12 mo	ICD	ICD mechanical complications	4.2%	--	--		
				ICD revision procedure	2.2%	--			
Gradaus, 2003 12914630	2,554	2.6 mo	Single- or dual-chamber ICD	ICD dislocation	1.9%	--	Lead dislocation	1.4%	--
MacFadden, 2012 22312139	4,830	1.5 mo††	Single- or dual-chamber ICD or CRT-D	--			Lead replacement	1.0%††	--
							Lead repositioning, any	1.2%††	--
							Lead dislodgement, repositioned	0.6%††	--
							Lead dislodgement, not repositioned	2.5%††	--

AE=adverse event; CRT-D=cardiac resynchronization therapy-defibrillator; ESRD=end stage renal disease; ICD=implantable cardioverter–defibrillator; mo=month; PMID=PubMed ID; Pt-y=Patient-year; RV=right ventricular; y=year. For study name acronyms see Appendix Table 16.

* Generator and/or lead models noted if documented.

† Includes ICD arm of trials from Key Question 1 with ≥500 patients with ICDs.

‡ Likely patient overlap between Thijssen,2012 [22094073], Borleffs [19808497] and Van Rees [22352338]. All data from Leiden University Medical Center Cardiology Information System (EPD-Vision).

§ Implanted systems were manufactured by Biotronik, Medtronic, Boston Scientific/Guidant, and St. Jude Medical/Ventritex

|| Likely patient overlap between Brullmar. [22154315] and Ditchl [21678454].

¶ These analyses exclude patients receiving Sprint Fidelis or Riata leads.

** per 100 lead-years.

†† calculated

‡‡ Includes perforations (0.38%), dislodgements, electrical malfunctions and other lead-related AEs.

§§573 events in 561 patients

|||| Insulation damage, conductor fracture, impedance issues

¶¶ Sensing issues, elevated threshold, loss of capture, diaphragmatic simulation, High DFT, unclassified

*** 220 events in 210 patients. From figure.

††† Includes 44 lead failures among 1985 patients with Sprint Fidelis (1.5 per 100 pt-yrs.)

‡‡‡ Biotronik generators capable of automatic remote home monitoring (Lumax 300 DR-T (1.3%), Lumax 300 DR-T (1.3%), Lumax 300 VR-T (1.1%), Lumax 340 VR-T (1.1%), Lumax 340 DR-T (22.2%), Lumax 340 VR-T (11.9%), Lumos DR-T (33.9%), Lumos

C-43

Appendix Table 20. Late adverse events: Device- and lead-related adverse events in patients with advisory leads or devices

Study Author, Year PMID	N	Mean Followup	Device Type [Model]*	Device- or Lead-Related Adverse Events	%
Advisory Devices					
Sengupta, 2012 22314669	704	70 mo	Single- or dual-chamber ICD or CRT-D [Advisory]	Device malfunction	6.1% †
Advisory Leads					
Hauser, 2002 22396584	1,035	86 mo maximum	ICD [Fidelis leads 6931, 6948, 6949]	Lead failure	8.1%
Tzogias, 2012 22314669, US	971	46 mo	Single- or dual-chamber ICD or CRT-D [Fidelis 6949 leads]	Lead failure	7.1%
				Lead fracture leading to failure	6.8% ‡
Cheung, 2012 22923271	602	42 mo median	ICD [Fidelis leads models 6949, 6931, 6948]	Lead failure	8.4%
Birnie, 2012 22311781	3,169	41 mo median	ICD [Fidelis leads]	Lead failure	7.9%
RAFT Parkash, 2012 23159551	818	39 mo median	ICD or CRT-D [Fidelis leads]	Lead failure	5.5%§
				Lead fracture	1.65% per year
Morrison, 2011 21737019	1,030	34 mo	ICD or CRT-D [Fidelis leads 6931, 6948, 6949]	Lead survival: 87.0%‖	--
Brumberg, 2012 22519559	621	32 mo	Single- or dual-chamber ICD or CRT-D [Fidelis leads]	Lead malfunction	8.4% ‡

CRT-D=cardiac resynchronization therapy-defibrillator; ICD=implantable cardioverter–defibrillator; mo=month; PMID=PubMed ID.

* Generator and/or lead models noted if documented.
† 4.0% advisory-related malfunctions. Device malfunction is patients with non-advisory devices: 1.6% (see Appendix Table 18). P<0.001 advisory versus non-advisory devices.
‡ Calculated
§ Lead failure in patients with non-Fidelis leads: 0.2%. (see Appendix Table 18A). P<0.0001 Fidelis vs. non-Fidelis leads.
‖ Lead survival in patients with non-advisory leads: 98.7% (see Appendix Table 18A). P<0.001 advisory versus non-advisory leads.

Appendix Table 21. Late adverse events: Infection and deep vein thrombosis

Study Author, Year PMID	N	Mean Followup	Device Type [Model]*	Infection	%	/100 Pt-Y	Thrombosis	%
ICD arms from RCTs†								
SCD-HeFT Freudenberger, 2007 17485579	681‡	45.5 mo Median	Single-chamber ICD [Medtronic 7223]	--			Any thrombo-embolic event	2.9%
MADIT II Moss, 2002, 1190728¢	742	20 mo	ICD [Guidant]	Non-fatal infection requiring surgical intervention	0.7%	--	--	
Other Studies								
Thijssen,2012 22094073	3,194§	49 mo	Single- or dual-chamber ICD or CRT-D [Multiple||]	Infection requiring ICD replacement	3.7%	--	--	
Bode, 2012 22753865	903	49 mo	ICD	--			Symptomatic subclavian venous thrombosis	0.9%
van Rees, 2012 22352338	1,602§	41 mo	ICD ¶	Infection (undefined)	2.7%		--	
Tsai, 2010 19262366	1,060	38 mo	ICD	Lead infection requiring antibiotics	0.5%	--	--	
Borleffs, 2009 19808497	2,068§	36 mo	Single- or dual-chamber ICD or CRT-D [Multiple||]	Pocket infection requiring lead removal	1.7%**	--	--	
De Bie, 2012 22056722	2,476§	30 mo median	ICD or CRT-D [Multiple||]	Infection requiring device and lead removal	2.6%	--	--	
Landolina, 2011 21576653	3,253	18 mo median	Single- or dual-chamber ICD or CRT-D [Medtronic]	Incisional infection treated conservatively	--	0.3%**	--	
				Infection requiring system removal	--	0.7%††		
Charytan, 2011 21664735	9,528 ESRD	16.8 mo**	ICD or CRT-D	Severe infection during 1st year ‡‡	--	98.8	--	
				Subsequent years (N=4,552)	--	63.9		
				Device infection	--	4.2		
Gradaus, 2003 12914630	1,033	12 mo	Single- or dual-chamber ICD	Infection of ICD device	0.9%**	--	--	
Remmelts, 2009 1932590	667	10 mo**	Single- or dual-chamber ICD or CRT-D	Pocket infection with or without bacteremia or ICD-related endocarditis	1.0%§§	1.2	--	
Lyman, 2011 21795298	38,992	3 mo	ICD	Infection	1.2%	--	Deep venous thrombosis	1.0%
Lee, 2010 20170816	3,340	1.5 mo	Single- or dual-chamber ICD or CRT-D	Pocket infection requiring debridement	1.0%	--	Subclavian venous thrombosis	0.2%
				Sepsis	0.2%	--		

CRT-D=cardiac resynchronization therapy-defibrillator; ESRD=end stage renal disease; ICD=implantable cardioverter-defibrillator; MADIT II=Multicenter Automatic Defibrillator Implantation Trial II; mo=month; PMID=PubMed ID; Pt-Y=patient-year; SCD-HeFT= Sudden Cardiac Death in Heart Failure Trial.

*   Generator and/or lead models noted if documented.

†   Includes ICD arm of trials from key question 1 with ≥500 patients with ICDs.

‡   Excludes patients with atrial fibrillation or flutter at baseline.

§   Likely patient overlap between Borleffs [19808497], de Bie [22056722], Thijssen [22094073] and Van Rees [22352338]. All data from Leiden University Medical Center Cardiology Information System (EPD-Vision).

‖   Implanted systems were manufactured by Biotronik, Medtronic, Boston Scientific/Guidant, and St. Jude Medical/Ventritex

¶   Excludes patients receiving Sprint Fidelis or Riata leads

**   Calculated

††   From figure

‡‡   Severe infection defined as any of the following: episodes coded as device infections, postoperative infections, bacteremia, septicemia, and all episodes in which patients received intravenous vancomycin.

§§   Data calculated. Includes N=2 (0.3%) post-operative infections.

Appendix Table 22. P values for comparisons of late adverse events and inappropriate shock by patient subgroup

Adverse Event	Primary vs. Secondary Prevention	LVEF	NYHA Class IV vs. III	Dual- vs. Single-chamber ICD	Single-chamber ICD vs. CRT-D	Age	Female*	DM	Lower Physician Volume	Lower Hospital Volume	OR vs. CCL
Inappropriate shocks	NS (A, E, F,U) P<0.001 (M) worse for secondary	NS (P)†	NS (P)	P=0.02 (C) worse for single-chamber NS (A, I)	NS (A)	P<0.01 (A), P<0.04 (K) P<0.05 (Q,M‡) nd (D) worse for younger	NS (A, M, O)	P=0.0076 (D) NS (J,M)	--	--	--
Surgical intervention / revision	NS (G§)‖	--	--	P=0.004 (H) worse for dual-chamber	P<0.001 (H) worse for CRT-D	--	--	--	NS (N)	P<0.01 (N)¶	--
Lead dislodgement, requiring intervention or undefined	NS (H**)	--	--	--	--	NS (H**,Q)	NS (H**, O§)	NS (J)	--	--	--
Lead dislodgement, no intervention	--	--	--	--	--	--	P=0.003 (O)	--	--	--	--
Lead malfunction / replacement / failure	--	--	--	--	--	NS (Q)	P<0.001 (O)	--	--	--	--
Recalled lead malfunction / failure	NS (R, S, T)	P=0.026 (R) worse for higher; NS (S, T, V)††	NS (V)	NS (L) NS (T)‡‡	P=0.0021 worse for CRT (V§§); NS (L, T‡‡)	P=0.016 worse for older (R); NS (L, T, V)	P=0.028 (L) P=0.005 (R) P=0.02 (S), NS (T, V)	NS (T)	--	--	--
Infection	NS (H)	--	--	nd (B§)	--	NS (H,Q)	NS (H,O§)	NS (H, J)	NS (N)	NS (N)	nd (B§)
Deep vein thrombosis	--	--	--	--	--	--	P=0.004 (O§)	--	P<0.01 (N)¶	NS (N)	--
Number of papers (reporting statistics)	10 (10)	5 (5)	2 (2)	7 (6)	5 (5)	10 (9)	9 (9)	5 (5)	1 (1)	1 (1)	1 (0)

A-R in parentheses indicate specific studies. (See Study Key, below)
P values <0.05 indicate statistically higher rates of AE in subgroup, unless otherwise noted. NS indicates no statistical difference in AE between subgroups. nd indicates paper reported rates of AE by subgroup but did not report statistical comparison between groups.

CCL=cardiac catheterization lab; CRT-D=cardiac resynchronization therapy-defibrillator; DM=diabetes mellitus; ICD=implantable cardioverter-defibrillator; LVEF=left ventricular ejection fraction; MADIT II=Multicenter Automatic Defibrillator Implantation Trial II; MADIT-CRT=Multicenter Automatic Defibrillator Implantation Trial with Cardiac Resynchronization Therapy; NYHA=New York Heart Association; OR=operating room; PMID=PubMed ID

* Adverse events are higher or NS different in females compared with males.
† LVEF 31-35% vs. ≤30%
‡ Paper reports hazard ratio with confidence interval that does not cross 1.0.
§ Less than 10 events in at least one subgroup.

|| Patients receiving ICDs for primary prevention compared with "other indications".

¶ Higher rates of AEs with lower ICD implantation volume.

** Left ventricular lead dislodgement in CRT-D patients

†† Worse for each 10% absolute increase in LVEF (R); not statistically significantly different for continuous LVEF (S, T) or LVEF >23% vs. ≤23% (V).

‡‡ No statistically significant difference across three subgroups: single-chamber ICD, dual-chamber ICD and CRT-D.

§§ Single- or dual-chamber ICD vs. CRT-D

<u>Study Key</u> (Author, Year, PMID)

A Van Rees, 2011, 21272746
B Remmelts, 2009, 19325900
C Larsen, 2010, 20186244
D Sandesara, 2011, 21086086
E Van Welsenes, 2011, 21208947
F Ditchl, 2011, 21678454
G Varma, 2010, 20716717

H Landolina, 2011, 21576653
I MADIT II, Berenbom, 2005, 16255753
J MADIT-CRT, Martin, 2011, 21350054
K Brullman, 2012, 22154315
L Brumberg, 2012, 22519559
M Kleemann, 2012, 2232331
N Lyman, 2011, 21795298

O McFadden, 2012, 22312139
P Sweeney, 2012, 22387371
Q van Rees, 2012, 21920909
R Birnie, 2012, 22311781
S Cheung, 2012, 22923271
T Tzogias, 2012, 22314669
U Sweeney, 2005, 15927965
V RAFT, Parkash, 2012, 23159551

Appendix Table 23. Eligibility criteria

Study Author, Year PMID Country	Study type (# of centers)	Total N (Study duration)	Inclusion							Specification regarding:			
			Age, y	Etiology	1° prevention	LVEF	NYHA	QRS interval	MI	Revascularization excluding CABG	CABG
Studies of patients with ischemic cardiomyopathy and remote MI (>30 or 40 days)											
ICD vs. no ICD											
MADIT Moss, 1996 8960472 US and EU	RCT (32)	196 (5 y; mean 27 mo)	25-80	Ischemic	Yes	≤35	I, II, III	nd	Inc: Q-wave or enzyme-positive MI ≥3 wk	Exc: Coronary angioplasty within the past 3 mo	Exc: CABG within the past 2 mo
MADIT II Moss, 2002 11907286 US and EU	RCT (76)	1232 (mean 20 mo; range 6 d–53 mo)	>21	Ischemic	Yes	≤30	I, II, III	nd	Inc: MI ≥1 mo Exc: MI within the past mo	Exc: Coronary revascularization within prior 3 mo	nd
Studies of patients with nonischemic cardiomyopathy											
ICD vs. no ICD											
AMIOVIRT Strickberger, 2003 12767651 US	RCT (10)	103 (5 y)	≥18	Nonischemic	Yes	≤35	I, II, III	nd	nd	nd	nd
CAT Bansch, 2002 11914254 Germany	RCT (15)	104 (6 y)	18-70	Nonischemic	Yes	≤30	II, III	nd	Exc: History of prior MI	nd	nd
DEFINITE Kadish, 2004 15152060 US	RCT (25)	458 (5 y; mean 2.4 y)	nd	Nonischemic	Yes	<36	I, II, III	nd	nd	nd	nd

Study Author, Year PMID Country	Study type (# of centers)	Total N (Study duration)	Inclusion						Specification regarding:		
			Age, y	Etiology	1° prevention	LVEF	NYHA	QRS interval	MI	Revascularization excluding CABG	CABG
Fonarow, 2000 10760339 US	Retrospective cohort (1)	147 (mean 22 mo)	nd	Nonischemic	Yes	<35	III, IV	nd	nd	nd	nd
Studies of patients with mixed ischemic and nonischemic cardiomyopathy **ICD vs. no ICD**											
Chan, 2009 20031808 US	Prospective cohort (7)	965 (5 y)	≥18	Ischemic, nonischemic	Yes	≤35	nd	>120 ms	Inc: MI of ≥30 d	nd	nd
COMPANION Bristow, 2004 15152059 US	RCT (128)	1520 (3.0 y; median 14 mo)	nd	Ischemic, nonischemic	Yes	≤35	III, IV	≥120 ms	nd	nd	nd
Mezu, 2011 21640321 US	Retrospective cohort (1)	152 (4 y; mean 2.3 y)	≥80	Ischemic, nonischemic	Yes	≤35	I, II, III (class I only if prior MI)	nd	nd	nd	nd
OPTIMIZE-HF and GWTG-HF Hernandez, 2010 20009044 US	Retrospective cohort, registry (nd)	4685 (3 y)	65-84	Ischemic, nonischemic	Yes	≤35	nd	nd	nd	nd	nd
SCD-HeFT Bardy, 2005 15659722 US	RCT (nd)	2521 (6 y; median 46 mo)	>18	Ischemic, nonischemic	Yes	≤35	II, III	nd	nd	nd	nd
ICD vs. CRT-D											
Diab, 2011 21700757 UK	RCT (1)	73 (6 mo)	nd	Ischemic, nonischemic	nd	≤35	III, IV	≥120 ms	nd	nd	nd

Study Author, Year PMID Country	Study type (# of centers)	Total N (Study duration)	Inclusion						Specification regarding:		
			Age, y	Etiology	1° prevention	LVEF	NYHA	QRS interval	MI	Revascularization excluding CABG	CABG
MADIT-CRT Moss, 2009 19723701 US, Canada, EU	RCT (110)	1820 (4 y; mean 2.4 y)	≥21	Ischemic, nonischemic	nd	≤30	I, II	≥130 ms	Exc: MI within 3 mo	Exc: PCI within 3 mo	Exc: Previous CABG within 3 mo
RAFT Tang 2010 21073365 Multi	RCT	1798 (mean 40 mo)	nd	Ischemic, nonischemic	nd (86% were primary prevention)	≤30	II, III	Intrinsic: ≥120 ms; Paced: ≥200ms	nd	nd	nd
Studies of patients with ischemic cardiomyopathy and recent MI (<30 days) or revascularization **ICD vs. no ICD**											
CABG-Patch Bigger, 1997 9371853 US and Germany	RCT (37)	900 (4 y; mean 2.7 y)	<80	Ischemic	Yes	<36	nd	≥114 ms	nd	nd	Inc: Scheduled for CABG Exc: Emergency CABG
DINAMIT Hohnloser, 2004 15590950 Multi	RCT (73)	674 (4 y; mean 2.5 y)	18-80	Ischemic	Yes	≤35	I, II, III	nd	Inc: MI (6-40 d prior)	Exc: 2-vessel PCI since the qualifying MI	Exc: CABG since the qualifying MI or planned within 4 wk
IRIS Steinbeck, 2009 19812399 Germany	RCT (nd)	898 (6 y; mean 37 mo)	18-80	Ischemic	Yes	≤40	I, II, III	nd	Inc: MI (5-31 d prior)	nd	Exc: An indication for CABG
ICD vs. CRT-D											

Study Author, Year PMID Country	Study type (# of centers)	Total N (Study duration)	Inclusion							Specification regarding:			
			Age, y	Etiology	1° prevention	LVEF	NYHA	QRS interval		MI	Revascularization excluding CABG	CABG
MENDMI Chung, 2010 20852059 US	RCT (29)	80 (12 mo)	nd	Ischemic	nd	≤35	I, II, III	<120 ms		Inc: Anterior MI 3-14 d	nd	Exc: CABG 30 d before or after enrollment

1°=primrary, CABG=coronary artery bypass graft, EU=Europe, ICD=implantable cardiac defibrillator, LVEF=left ventricular ejection fraction, MI=myocardial infarction, mo=month, ms=millisecond, nd=not documented, NYHA=New York Heart Association, RCT=randomized controlled trial, UK, United Kingdom, US=United States, wk=week, y=year
For study names, see Appendix Table 1.

www.ingramcontent.com/pod-product-compliance
Lightning Source LLC
Chambersburg PA
CBHW080245180526
45167CB00006B/2426